Companion for

1st MBBS

Companion for
1st MBBS

Includes the Latest CBME-based Question Papers

17th Edition

Singi Yatiraj
Kalaburagi, Karnataka
India

Co-author
Roopali Somani
Kalaburagi, Karnataka
India

JAYPEE

JAYPEE BROTHERS MEDICAL PUBLISHERS
The Health Sciences Publisher
New Delhi | London

JAYPEE **Jaypee Brothers Medical Publishers (P) Ltd**

Headquarters
EMCA House
23/23-B, Ansari Road, Daryaganj
New Delhi 110 002, India
Landline: +91-11-23272143, +91-11-23272703
+91-11-23282021, +91-11-23245672
E-mail: jaypee@jaypeebrothers.com

Corporate Office
Jaypee Brothers Medical Publishers (P) Ltd.
4838/24, Ansari Road, Daryaganj
New Delhi 110 002, India
Phone: +91-11-43574357
Fax: +91-11-43574314
E-mail: jaypee@jaypeebrothers.com

Overseas Office
JP Medical Ltd.
83, Victoria Street, London
SW1H 0HW (UK)
Phone: +44-20 3170 8910
Fax: +44(0)20 3008 6180
E-mail: info@jpmedpub.com

Website: www.jaypeebrothers.com

Website: www.jaypeedigital.com

Inquiries for bulk sales may be solicited at: jaypee@jaypeebrothers.com

Companion for 1st MBBS

First Edition : *2005*
Second Edition : *2007*
Third Edition : *2008*
Fourth Edition : *2009*
Fifth Edition : *2010*
Sixth Edition : *2011*
Seventh Edition : *2012*
Eighth Edition : *2013*
Ninth Edition : *2014*
Tenth Edition : *2015*
Eleventh Edition : *2016*
Twelfth Edition : *2016*
Thirteenth Edition : 2017
Fourteenth Edition : 2018
Fifteenth Edition : 2019
Sixteenth Edition : 2020
Seventeenth Edition : 2021
Revised Reprint : **2025**

ISBN 978-93-5465-497-8

Printed at: Sterling Graphics Pvt. Ltd.

|| ऊँ श्री फलौदी ब्रम्हाणी देवी नमः ||

Om Shri Falaudi Brahmani Devi Namah

Dedicated to

That person
Who has brought happiness in my life
Who has given me a reason to smile
Who has trusted me all the time and
Showed me that I can do it.

This book is a tribute to my
Late Sister Anupama
and
Grandmother Rajubai

PREFACE

Dear Students,

In the competitive market of question banks, there was a vacant slot for an exclusive, original, authentic, and updated question bank, which is being filled today by this book.

This book has all the ingredients for success in the university examination. It has the original questions of the Rajiv Gandhi University of Health Sciences (RGUHS), Karnataka, India, course contents prescribed by the university. The questions are arranged chapterwise and references given from the latest editions of the commonly read student-popular books. The most important aspect of this question bank is its originality, i.e., the questions asked in the paper are kept the same way without major alterations so that students can get an idea about the various ways of asking the same question.

Short answer questions form the mainstay of scoring in the examination and this is the only question bank, which has given them their due importance. They have been classified exclusively and given cross-reference for easy reading during peak examination time.

This book has questions from RGUHS only. It does not deal with previous universities because they had different marking schemes, which are outdated. It is questions of RGUHS that get repeated in the university examination and again this is the first book that has questions from RGUHS only.

Students will find the questions well-classified and easy-to-read because cross-references are from the latest editions that most students possess.

I hope, this book will be well received by the student fraternity and it will serve the purpose it is meant for. Any queries and comments are welcome.

I sincerely solicit your valuable comments in this regard. So please do write your comments to my mail *singi_yatiraj@yahoo.com* or in Facebook on my page *Singi Yatiraj.*

Wishing you all the best.

Singi Yatiraj
singi_yatiraj@yahoo.com

ACKNOWLEDGMENTS

I would like to thank:

- Dr B Mallikarjun, Former Dean, MR Medical College, Kalaburagi, Karnataka, India, for his encouragement and support.
- All the staff members of Department of Anatomy, Physiology and Biochemistry, MR Medical College, Kalaburagi, for their selfless excellent teaching.
- My teachers, for they are the ones who made me this capable.
- My friends Kiran, Nagaraj and Wali, for their help, support, suggestions and encouragement throughout the project.
- Mr Kalburgi and *Late* Mr Puranik of Computer Section, for providing me the question papers of the recent university examinations.
- All the students who have helped me compile the question bank.
- Mr Md Bari, Mr Yousuf Patel and Mr Rashid, Star Computers, for all the timely assistance and neat computer printing of the manuscript.
- Mr Suresh Prithvi, Proprietor, M/s Prithvi Books Agency and his staff, for their support, cooperation and promoting this title. Mr Santosh Patil, Proprietor, M/s SS Patil Book Sellers and staff, for their cooperation.
- My all friends and well-wishers, for their best wishes.
- Shri Jitendar P Vij (Group Chairman), Mr Ankit Vij (Managing Director), Mr MS Mani (Group President), Dr Madhu Choudhary (Director–Educational Publishing), Ms Pooja Bhandari [Director–Production (Books and Journals)], Mr Ajay Kumar Sharma [Deputy General Manager (Books and Journals)], Ms Sunita Katla (Executive Assistant to Group Chairman and Publishing Manager) of M/s Jaypee Brothers Medical Publishers (P) Ltd, New Delhi, India, for publishing the book in the same format as wanted well in time.
- Mr Venugopal (Associate Director–South) and other staff members of Jaypee Brothers, Bengaluru Branch, for taking this book to every corner of Karnataka.
- Dr Upma Tomar (Sr Development Editor), Ms Samina Khan (Executive Assistant to Director–Educational Publishing), Mr Vijay Kumar Bhatia (Manager–Production), Ms Seema Dogra (Cover Visualizer), Ms Neha Verma (Graphic Designer–Cover), Ms Uma Adhikari (Typesetter), Ms Geeta Rani (Proofreader) and others at the M/s Jaypee Brothers Medical Publishers (P) Ltd, New Delhi, for their painstaking effort to make this book attractive and lucid.
- All the students, for their overwhelming response and support to my prior endeavors.

- All those who have helped me directly or indirectly.
- Most important of all, my parents, sister, uncles, aunties and cousins, for their eternal love, care and support.
- Last but not least, a very special and sincere thanks to my loving sister Roopali Somani, for sharing the burden of my heavy workload by helping me out with Companion series.

Thank you all of you,

Without you, this book would not have been a reality.

CONTENTS

ANATOMY

PHYSIOLOGY

BIOCHEMISTRY

1

ANATOMY

REFERENCES

1. Krishna Garg **(BDCGA)**: BD Chaurasia's Handbook of General Anatomy (7th Edition), CBS Publishers & Distributors, New Delhi, ₹ 369/-
2. V Subhadra Devi **(VSDGA)**: Textbook of General Anatomy (2nd Edition), Jaypee: The Health Science Publishers, New Delhi, ₹ 525/-
3. BD Chaurasia **(BDC Vol: 1)**: Human Anatomy, Volume One (10th Edition), CBS Publishers & Distributors, New Delhi, ₹ 831/-
4. BD Chaurasia **(BDC Vol: 2)**: Human Anatomy, Volume Two (10th Edition), CBS Publishers & Distributors, New Delhi, ₹ 894/-
5. BD Chaurasia **(BDC Vol: 3 & 4)**: Human Anatomy, Volume Three (10th Edition), CBS Publishers & Distributors, New Delhi, ₹ 1776/- (Inclusive of Volume 4)
6. Raveendranath Veeramani (IBSEMB): Inderbir Singh's Human Embryology (14th Edition), Jaypee: The Health Science Publishers, New Delhi, ₹ 995/-
7. Pushpalatha K, Deepa Bhat & Pushpa NB **(IBSHST)**: Inderbir Singh's Textbook of Human Histology (11th Edition), Jaypee: The Health Science Publishers, New Delhi, ₹ 895/-
8. V Subhadra Devi **(IBSANT1)**: Inderbir Singh's Textbook of Anatomy, Volume One (7th Edition), Jaypee: The Health Science Publishers, New Delhi, ₹ 795/-
9. V Subhadra Devi **(IBSANT2)**: Inderbir Singh's Textbook of Anatomy, Volume Two (7th Edition), Jaypee: The Health Science Publishers, New Delhi, ₹ 795/-
10. V Subhadra Devi **(IBSANT3)**: Inderbir Singh's Textbook of Anatomy, Volume Three (7th Edition), Jaypee: The Health Science Publishers, New Delhi, ₹ 795/-
11. DK Kadasne **(KDSN)**: Textbook of Embryology (1st Edition), Jaypee: The Health Science Publishers, New Delhi, ₹ 495/-
12. Victor P. Eroschenko **(DFIOR)**: diFiore's Atlas of Histology (13th Edition), Wolter Kluwer, ₹ 775/-

ANATOMY

Curriculum

	BDCGA	VSDGA	

SECTION 1: GENERAL ANATOMY

CHAPTER 1: INTRODUCTION

Short Answer

1. Four important criteria of anatomical position of the human body.	11	5	D01

CHAPTER 2: SKELETON

Short Essays

1. Classify the bones and explain the components of the long bone.	48, 62	65	J14
2. Classification of bones.	48	65	D16
3. Sesamoid bone.	54	65	D03
4. Epiphyses—definition, types and examples.	62	56	D09(RS2), J05, J08
5. Blood supply of a long bone.	65	60	D06, J11

Short Answers

1. Classification of bones.	48	65	J99
2. Define pneumatic bones with example. Mention its functional significance.	53	65	J98
3. Sesamoid bone—features, examples.	54	65	J19(RS3), D00, J06, D09, J12
4. Name the types of lamellae in compact bone.	58	64	D02
5. Growing end of long bone.	62	56	D05(RS2)
6. What are the types of epiphysis? Define each with example.	62	56	J98, J01, D04
7. Epiphysis.	62	56	J07(RS2), J14(RS3), D98
8. Metaphysis.	63	59	D98
9. Atavastic epiphysis.	63	58	J03
10. Traction epiphysis.	63	58	D03
11. Blood supply of long bone.	65	60	D07(RS2)

Contd...

Contd...

	BDCGA	VSDGA	
12. Laws of ossification.	68	69	J11(RS2), D99, J00, J04
13. Types of cartilages with examples.	73	56	J15
14. What are the features of fibro-cartilage?	74	56	D06(RS2)

CHAPTER 3: JOINTS

Short Essays

1. Classification of joints.	85	100	J08(RS2)
2. Classify joints. Discuss the components of the synovial joints.	85, 96	100, 106	D13
3. Classification of cartilaginous joints.	94	106	J98
4. Features of a typical synovial joint.	96	106	J05(RS2), J09

Short Answers

1. Bursa and its functions.	—	109	J06(RS2), J00, D00
2. Classify fibrous joints and give examples for each.	89	103	J14
3. Fibrous joint (types).	89	101	D15(RS3), J99, J10
4. Sutural joints.	89	103	D08
5. Syndesmosis.	91	103	J07, J09
6. Cartilaginous joint.	92	105	D12(RS3), N20(RS3)
7. Synchondrosis (primary cartilaginous joint).	92	106	D07
8. Symphysis (secondary cartilaginous joint).	93	106	J08
9. Define symphysis and give any two examples.	93	106	D11
10. Structural features of typical synovial joint.	96	106	J07, D07
11. Classify synovial joint with examples of each type.	96	112	J13(RS3), J01, D04

Contd...

Contd...

	BDCGA	VSDGA	
12. Name any two hinge joints.	96	112	J06
13. Mention two examples of pivot joints.	96	112	D05
14. Hilton's law.	109	—	J03
Multiple Choice Questions			
1. Which one of the following is not a synovial joint? a. Pivot b. Saddle c. Ellipsoid d. **Syndesmosis**	96	103	J21(RS4)

CHAPTER 4: MUSCLES

Short Answers

1. What is the difference between a multipennate muscle and a strap muscle?	—	—	D05
2. Give the types of pinnate muscles with one example of each.	131	93	D10, D14
3. Bipennate muscle.	131	93	D07
4. Prime movers with examples.	145	94	J17(RS3)

CHAPTER 5: CARDIOVASCULAR SYSTEM

Short Answers

1. Collateral circulation.	—	135	J14(RS3), D08
2. Name various types of capillaries and sites where they are present.	166	132	D10(RS2), D07
3. Anastomoses—three types with suitable examples.	168	135	F21(RS4)
4. End arteries—definition and examples.	172	137	D16(RS3), D06, J08, D15

CHAPTER 6: LYMPHATIC SYSTEM

None

Contd...

ANATOMY

Contd...

	BDCGA	VSDGA	
CHAPTER 7: NERVOUS SYSTEM			
Long Essay			
1. Draw and label a typical spinal nerve. What is its distribution and applied anatomy?	—	169	J00
Short Answers			
1. Define a spinal segment.	—	169	D99, D06, J08
2. Draw and label part of a multipolar neurons.	207	162	D05(RS2), D99, J04
3. Give any four differences between axon and dendrite.	207	—	J01, D02, D04
4. Classify neurons according to their structure with suitable examples.	207	158	J21(RS4), D03
5. Name any two types of synapses and two neurotransmitters.	208	164	D00
6. Mention the types of neuroglia giving examples.	209	164	J02, D06
CHAPTER 8: SKIN AND FASCIAE			
Short Essay			
1. Interosseous membrane.	257	46	J08(RS2)
Short Answers			
1. Enumerate any three modifications of the deep fascia in the body with suitable examples from the upper limb.	255	45	J21(RS4)
2. Name the appendages of skin.	244	39	D01, J06
3. Give any six functions of skin.	249	34	D11
4. Enumerate the functions of interosseous membrane.	257	46	D11
CHAPTER 9: CONNECTIVE TISSUE, LIGAMENTS AND RAPHE			
Short Answers			
1. Name the components of the connective tissue.	263	26	J13
2. Connective tissue fibers.	264	26	D18(RS3)

Contd...

Contd...

	BDCGA	VSDGA	
3. Name the types of connective tissues giving examples.	264	29	D00
4. Cells of connective tissue.	264	27	J11(RS2)

	BDC Vol:1	IBSANT1	

SECTION 2: UPPER LIMB

CHAPTER 10: INTRODUCTION

None.

CHAPTRER 11: BONES OF UPPER LIMB

Short Essays

1. Coracoid process of scapula.	11	17	D01
2. Upper end of humerus.	13	22	J06(RS2)

Short Answers

1. Mention peculiarities of the clavicle.	6	12	J98, D99
2. Muscles attached to clavicle.	8	13	J05
3. Name ligaments attached to clavicle.	8	13	J02
4. Coracoid process.	11	17	J15(RS3), D18(RS3)
5. Name muscles attached to medial border of scapula.	11	19	D00
6. Attachments to coracoid process of scapula.	11	20	J00, J01, D04, D05, J11, D16
7. Bicipital groove of humerus and structures attached.	13	23	J98, J05, D06, J08, D08
8. Surgical neck of humerus and structures related to it.	13	23	D05(RS2), J06
9. Radial groove (spiral groove).	14	25	J99, D03
10. Name the muscles arising from posterior surface of shaft of ulna.	22	44	D08
11. Name the carpal bones.	23	46	J13(RS3)

Contd...

ANATOMY

Contd...

	BDC Vol:1	IBSANT1	
12. Pisiform bone.	23	49	D02

CHAPTER 12: PECTORAL REGION

Long Essay

1. Describe the female mammary gland under the following headings: (a) Extent/position; (b) Structure; (c) Relations; (d) Blood supply; (e) Lymphatic drainage; (f) Nerve supply; (g) Applied anatomy; (h) Development.	32	132	J09(RS2), D14(RS3), J15(RS3), D18(RS3)

Short Essays

1. Mammary gland—blood supply, lymphatic drainage and applied anatomy.	32	132	D06(RS2), J08(RS2), J17(RS3), D17(RS3), J19(RS3), D98, D07
2. Pectoralis major.	38	128	D14(RS3), D19(RS3)
3. Pectoralis minor.	38	128	D13(RS3), D17(RS3)
4. Clavipectoral fascia—extent, attachments and structures piercing it.	39	126	J07(RS2), D11(RS3), J13(RS3), J19(RS3), J99, J00, J06
5. Serratus anterior—attachments, nerve supply and actions.	41	128	J10(RS2), D02, D05, D14

Short Answers

1. Retromammary space.	32	133	D06
2. Peau d'orange.	36	141	D09
3. Clavipectoral fascia	39	126	J11(RS2)
4. Structures piercing clavipectoral fascia.	39	126	D00, J03, D06, D08, J10
5. Winging of scapula and how it is produced?	41	132	J98

Contd...

Contd...

	BDC Vol:1	IBSANT1	
Multiple Choice Questions			
1. True statement regarding pectoralis major muscle is: a. It is quadrilateral in shape b. **Inserted to lateral lip of bicipital groove** c. Divides axillary artery into three parts d. Clavicular head originates from lateral 1/3rd of anterior surface of clavicle.	38	128	J21(RS4)
CHAPTER 13: AXILLA			
Long Essays			
1. Describe the axillary artery under the following headings: (a) Beginning and termination; (b) Relations; (c) Branches; (d) Applied anatomy.	46	88	J07(RS2), D01, J15
2. Describe the brachial plexus under the following headings: (a) Formation; (b) Parts (roots, trunks, cords); (c) Relations; (d) Branches and distribution; (e) Applied anatomy. Add a note on carpal tunnel syndrome/add a note on Erb's paralysis/Explain the anatomical basis of the winging of the scapula.	52	56	J21(RS4), D06(RS2), J08(RS2), J12(RS3), D15(RS3), J10, D99, D03, D11, D15
Short Essays			
1. Axillary artery—extent, relations and branches.	46	88	J10(RS2), J11(RS2), D09
2. Axillary lymph nodes.	51	117	J11, D14
3. Describe the formation and branching pattern of the brachial plexus.	52	56	D08, D13
4. Lateral cord of brachial plexus.	54	58	D06
5. Erb's point and its applied anatomy (Erb-Duchenne's paralysis).	55	63	J05(RS2), J14(RS3), D19(RS3), D98, D09
Short Answers			
1. Structures forming anterior wall of axilla.	45	145	D05

Contd...

ANATOMY

Contd...

	BDC Vol:1	IBSANT1	
2. Contents of axilla.	46	146	J10(RS2)
3. Branches of axillary artery (2nd part and 3rd part).	50	88	J05(RS2), J01, D04, D05, J06, D13
4. Long thoracic nerve.	54	61	J06
5. Branches of medial cord of brachial plexus.	54	60	D00, J14, J15
6. Branches of posterior cord of the brachial plexus.	55	60	D16(RS3)
7. Erbs point—formation.	55	63	J13(RS3), D16
8. Erb's paralysis.	55	63	J01, D04
9. Klumpke's paralysis.	55	67	J08

CHAPTER 14: BACK

Short Essays

1. Trapezius muscle.	59	155	D14(RS3)
2. Rhomboideus major muscle.	59	156	D17(RS3)

Short Answer

1. Nerve supply and actions of trapezius muscle.	59	155	J12(RS3), J03

CHAPTER 15: SCAPULAR REGION

Long Essay

1. Describe the root value, formation course, relations and branches of axillary nerve. Give its applied anatomy. What are effects of injury at surgical neck of humerus?	71	73	J99, D07

Short Essays

1. Deltoid muscle—location, attachments, nerve supply and action.	64	158	J08(RS2), D13(RS3), D18(RS3), J00, D01, J05, J06
2. Structures undercover of deltoid muscle.	66	159	J16(RS3), J18(RS3)

Contd...

ANATOMY

Contd...

	BDC Vol:1	IBSANT1	
3. A 30-year-old cricketer felt moderate pain in the right shoulder for the last two weeks. The pain was severe enough to prevent him from bowling. He visited a sports medicine specialist who observed that maximum pain was felt in the mid-range abduction. A diagnosis of rotator cuff tendinitis was a made: a. Describe the components of the rotator cuff b. Explain the functional importance of the rotator cuff c. Explain the anatomical basis for the maximum pain felt in the mid-range of abduction	64	163	F21(RS4)
4. Rotator cuff of shoulder.	64	163	J15(RS3), D10, J15
5. Describe the boundaries and contents of the intermuscular spaces in the upper limb (quadrangular and triangular spaces).	64	167	J09(RS2), J02, D04, J07, D13
6. Axillary nerve (circumflex nerve).	71	73	J14(RS3), N20(RS3), J98, J12
7. Anastomosis around scapula.	70	92	J12
Short Answers			
1. Nerve supply and action of deltoid.	67	159	D03, J13
2. Rotator cuff (muscles forming it).	64	163	J09(RS2), J18(RS3), D16
3. Boundaries and contents of the inferior triangular intermuscular space in the arm.	71	168	D11(RS3), J14
4. Axillary nerve in relation to surgical neck of humerus.	71	73	D14(RS3)

CHAPTER 16: CUTANEOUS NERVES, SUPERFICIAL VEINS AND LYMPHATIC DRAINAGE

Short Essays

1. Venous drainage of upper limb.	77	109	D06
2. Cephalic vein.	78	109	J12(RS3)

Contd...

ANATOMY

Contd...

	BDC Vol:1	IBSANT1	
Short Answers			
1. Supraclavicular nerve.	73	55	D05
2. Cutaneous innervation of dorsum of hand.	75	237	J98, J03
3. Cutaneous nerve supply of ring finger—diagram only.	75	—	D15(RS3)
4. Cephalic vein.	78	109	J13(RS3), D13(RS3), D17(RS3)
5. Basilic vein—commencement, termination and tributaries.	78	110	D99
6. Median cubital vein—connection and applied importance.	79	111	J18(RS3), D19(RS3), D13, D15
7. A 30-year-old lady had to get blood drawn for some routine blood tests. At the hospital laboratory, the technician selected a vein that ran across the roof of the cubital fossa for the collection of blood. a. Which vein did the technician select for drawing blood? b. Explain the anatomical basis for the selection of this vein	79	111	F21(RS4)
8. Explain the anatomical basis for selecting the median cubital vein for venepuncture.	79	111	J21(RS4)

CHAPTER 17: ARM

Long Essay			
1. Describe the origin, root value, course, relations, branches and applied anatomy of radial nerve (till it reaches elbow).	97	76	D00, J02, J04, D05
Short Essays			
1. Musculocutaneous nerve—root value, origin, relations, course, branches and termination. Explain why the motor distribution of the musculocutaneous nerve is affected in Erb's palsy.	87	68	F21(RS4), J08, J09, J10

Contd...

Contd...

	BDC Vol:1	IBSANT1	
2. Biceps brachii muscle—attachments, nerve supply and actions.	86	181	D05(RS2), D99, J08
3. Brachial artery.	89	95	J06(RS2), D02, J07
4. Anastomosis around elbow joint.	91	98	D06(RS2), D99
5. Cubital fossa—boundaries and contents.	92	188	J07(RS2), D09(RS2), J16(RS3), D98, J08
Short Answers			
1. Musculocutaneous nerve (muscles supplied).	87	68	J11(RS2), D11
2. Coracobrachialis.	86	181	J15
3. Biceps brachii muscle (attachments, nerve supply and actions).	86	181	J14
4. Brachialis—attachments, nerve supply and action.	86	181	J04
5. Branches of brachial artery.	90	96	D03
6. Events at insertion of coracobrachialis.	102	182	J00
7. Cubital fossa—boundaries, contents and clinical applications (neat labeled diagram).	92	188	D12(RS3), J99, J05, J06, D10, D14
8. Radial nerve in spiral groove.	97	76	D17(RS3)
9. Saturday night palsy.	98	80	J04, J05, D05
10. Wrist drop.	98	80	D06(RS2), D99, J03, J06
11. Branches of profunda brachii artery.	99	97	J09
CHAPTER 18: FOREARM AND HAND			
Long Essays			
1. Describe the ulnar nerve in the palm under the following headings: (a) Root value; (b) Relations; (c) Branches of distribution; (d) Applied anatomy.	124	70	J05(RS2), D14
2. Name the spaces in the palm. Describe the boundaries of midpalmar space. Add a note on its applied anatomy.	130	230	D09(RS2)

Contd...

Contd...

	BDC Vol:1	IBSANT1	
Short Essays			
1. Flexor digitorum superficialis muscle.	104	199	J02, D04
2. Radial artery—origin, termination, course, relations and branches.	107	100	D05, J14
3. Flexor retinaculum of hand.	113	220	D05(RS2), D12(RS3), D15(RS3), D99
4. Palmar aponeurosis.	114	223	N20(RS3), J00
5. Lumbricals—attachments, nerve supply, action and applied importance.	116	229	D16(RS3), D18(RS3), J04, J13, D16
6. Interossei of hand.	116	229	J13(RS3)
7. Superficial palmar arch—position, formation and branches.	122	104	D13(RS3), J14
8. Deep palmar arch.	123	105	D10
9. Ulnar nerve in hand.	124	70	J06(RS2), J18(RS3), D98
10. Median nerve in palm (hand).	125	83	J10(RS2), D10(RS2)
11. Carpal tunnel syndrome.	127	84	J01, D08, D11
12. Boundaries and contents of the midpalmar space.	130	231	D05
13. Thenar space.	130	232	J19(RS3)
14. Anatomical snuff box—boundaries and contents.	132	241	D09, D11
15. Extensor reticulum of wrist/hand.	133	239	J10(RS2), D10(RS2), J18(RS3), J07
16. Supinator muscle.	137	214	D09(RS2)
17. Posterior interosseous nerve.	138	76	J01
Short Answers			
1. Pronator teres muscles.	104	199	J99

Contd...

ANATOMY

Contd...

	BDC Vol:1	IBSANT1	
2. Flexor digitorum profundus—nerve supply and action.	105	202	D09
3. Anterior interosseous artery.	109	104	J16(RS3)
4. Flexor reticulum of hand—attachments/structures passing superficial/structures passing deep (through carpal tunnel).	113	220	J09(RS2), J10(RS2), J11(RS2), J19(RS3), J00, D00, J05, J09, D12, D14, J15, D15
5. Palmar aponeurosis.	114	223	J11(RS2), J13(RS3), J16(RS3)
6. Dupuytren's contracture.	115	225	D06
7. Name the hypothenar muscles and their nerve supply.	116	227	D15
8. Muscles of hypothenar eminence.	116	227	J05(RS2), D08(RS2)
9. Adductor pollicis.	116	227	D12(RS3), J15(RS3)
10. Lumbricals of hand—nerve supply, actions.	116	229	J06(RS2), J08(RS2), D11(RS3), J05, D10, J11, D13
11. Nerve supply of dorsal interossei of hand.	117	229	J10
12. Superficial palmar arch.	122	104	D08(RS2)
13. Deep palmar arch.	123	105	D07(RS2)
14. Claw hand.	125	73	D09(RS2), J11(RS2), D02, J04
15. Ulnar claw hand.	125	73	D12
16. Median nerve in carpal tunnel.	125	83	D13(RS3), J16(RS3), D19(RS3)
17. Carpal tunnel syndrome	127	84	N20(RS3)
18. Fascial spaces of hand.	129	230	D06(RS2)

Contd...

Contd...

	BDC Vol:1	IBSANT1	
19. Midpalmar space.	130	231	D05(RS2)
20. Anatomical snuff box.	132	241	J17(RS3)
21. Dorsal digital expansions—components.	136	242	J17(RS3), J00, D02, D15
22. Posterior interosseous artery.	139	104	D14(RS3)

CHAPTER 19: JOINTS OF UPPER LIMB

Long Essays

1. Describe the shoulder joint under the following headings: (a) Type and subtype; (b) Formation/articular ends; (c) Capsule and ligaments; (d) Relations; (e) Movements and muscles producing them; (f) Blood supply; (g) Nerve supply. Add a note on applied anatomy.	143	252	J10(RS2), D12(RS3), D16(RS3), J17(RS3), J01, J03, J11, J12, D12, J13, D16
2. Describe the elbow joint under the following headings: (a) Formation; (b) Ligaments; (c) Movements; (d) Blood supply; (e) Applied anatomy.	148	266	J16(RS3)
3. Describe the first carpometacarpal joint of hand.	158	281	D10(RS2)

Short Essays

1. Describe the movements of the scapula and the muscles causing them. Explain the anatomical basis of winging of the scapula.	41	132, 165	F21(RS4), J07(RS2)
2. Describe the articular surfaces, ligaments, movements of the shoulder joint.	143	252	J14
3. Abduction and adduction movements at shoulder joint.	146	261	D06
4. Elbow joint.	148	266	N20(RS3)
5. Radioulnar joints.	153	271	J09(RS2), J98, D03
6. Describe the articulation of the proximal radioulnar joint. Explain the movements and muscles causing the movements at this joint.	153	272	J21(RS4)

Contd...

Contd...

	BDC Vol:1	IBSANT1	
7. Supination and pronation.	154	276	D08(RS2), J11(RS2), J18(RS3), D02, J10
8. Movements of wrist joint.	157	278	D07(RS2), D11(RS3)
9. First carpometacarpal joint of thumb.	158	281	J07
10. Movements of thumb and muscles producing them.	158	283	D08, J09
Short Answers			
1. Coracoclavicular ligament.	141	248	D09(RS2)
2. Coracoacrominal arch—attachments and functions.	143	256	D06(RS2)
3. Glenohumeral ligaments.	143	255	D07(RS2), J12(RS3)
4. Movements of shoulder joint.	146	259	D19(RS3)
5. Radioulnar joint.	153	271	D07(RS2)
6. Functions of interosseous membrane.	154	275	D99
7. Muscles responsible for pronation and supination supinators and pronators) and their nerve supply.	154	276	D00, D15
8. Muscles supinating forearm with their nerve supply.	154	276	D07

CHAPTER 20: MISCELLANEOUS

Long Essays			
1. Describe the formation, branches, distribution and applied anatomy of median nerve.	125	81	D10
2. Describe the origin, course, relations and distribution of the ulnar nerve. Add a note on its applied anatomy (related to its damage in forearm).	124	68	J06
Short Answer			
1. Root value and muscles supplied by the radial nerve.	112	76	J14(RS3)

Contd...

Contd...

	BDC Vol:1	IBSANT1	
SECTION 3: THORAX			
CHAPTER 21: INTRODUCTION			
Short Essays			
1. Sternal angle—location, events occurring, clinical importance.	181	335	J04, J07, J12
2. Suprapleural membrane.	184	300	D07(RS2)
Short Answers			
1. Sternal angle—its importance and events occurring.	181	335	J06(RS2), D06(RS2), J11(RS2), D13(RS3), J18(RS3), D19(RS3), J98, D02
2. Suprapleural membrane (Sibson's fascia)—attachments.	184	300	J13(RS3), N20(RS3), J07, D16
CHAPTER 22: BONES AND JOINTS OF THORAX			
Short Essay			
1. First rib.	195	338	D06(RS2)
Short Answers			
1. Xiphisternal joint.	—	350	D16
2. First rib (peculiarities/atypical features, structures related).	195	338	J07(RS2), J15(RS3), J17(RS3), J03
3. Cervical rib.	198	343	D09
4. Name the muscles attached to sternum.	198	332	J15
5. Identify features of typical thoracic vertebra.	199	327	D03, D06, J13
CHAPTER 23: WALLS OF THORAX			
Long Essays			
1. Describe course, branches and distribution of typical intercostal nerve.	208	369	J07(RS2)

Contd...

Contd...

	BDC Vol:1	IBSANT1	
2. Describe a typical intercostal space under the following headings: (a) Definition; (b) Boundaries; and (c) Contents. Explain where needle is inserted into the intercostal space to drain a pleural effusion and the anatomical basis for the same. Name the structures in order from the skin to the pleura that must be pierced in order to enter the pleural cavity.	210, 246	357	F21(RS4)
Short Essays			
1. First intercostal space.	—	—	J03
2. Typical intercostal nerve—course, relations and branches.	208	369	J05(RS2), J17(RS3), D06, D00
3. Define a typical intercostal space. Describe the boundaries and contents of a typical intercostals space.	210	357	J21(RS4), D08(RS2), J16(RS3), D18(RS3), J08, J15
4. Azygos system of veins—definition, labeled diagram and applied anatomy.	214	377	D05
5. Azygos vein (vena azygous).	214	377	D10(RS2), D13(RS3), D14(RS3), J99, J09, D14
Short Answers			
1. Superior intercostal artery.	—	375	J09
2. Anterior intercostal membrane.	207	359	J11
3. External intercostal muscle.	207	360	J08(RS2)
4. Typical intercostal nerve (branches).	208	369	D06(RS2), J13
5. Contents of a typical intercostal space.	210	357	D98, D16
6. Enumerate the contents of coastal groove with their relations (order and name of structures in costal groove).	210	303	D99, D14

Contd...

Contd...

	BDC Vol:1	IBSANT1	
7. Azygos vein—level, formation, termination and tributaries.	214	377	D02, J11, D11, J15

CHAPTER 24: THORACIC CAVITY AND PLEURAE

Short Essays

1. Pleura.	223	408	D10
2. Pleural recesses—location, events occurring, clinical importance.	226	415	J07(RS2), J12(RS3), D16(RS3), J98, J04, D12

Short Answers

1. Pulmonary ligament and its function.	226	411	D12(RS3), J19(RS3), D99, D06
2. Pleural recess and its role.	226	415	J03
3. Costodiaphragmatic recess.	226	415	D19(RS3), D16

CHAPTER 25: LUNGS

Long Essays

1. Describe the lungs under the following headings: (a) Labeled diagram of mediastinal surfaces showing position of related structures including structures in both hila; (b) Development; (c) One congenital malformation.	230	420	D05
2. Define bronchopulmonary segments. Name the bronchopulmonary segments present in the left lung and add a note on its applied aspects. Draw a labeled diagram of the medial surfaces of both lungs.	238	430	D05(RS2)

Short Essays

1. Right lung.	230	420	D12(RS3)
2. Mediastinal surface of left lung with the aid of diagram.	232	428	D07(RS2), D10(RS2), J99
3. Mediastinal surface of right lung with the aid of diagram.	232	428	J08(RS2), J06

Contd...

Contd...

	BDC Vol:1	IBSANT1	
4. Mediastinal surface of lung.	232	428	D18(RS3)
5. Root of right lung—relations and structures forming it.	233	427	D06(RS2)
6. Hilum of lungs.	233	427	D00
7. List the differences between right and left lung.	235	429	J13
8. Bronchopulmonary segments (of left lung/of right lung).	238	430	J06(RS2), J11(RS2), D14(RS3), J17(RS3), D19(RS3), J00, J02, D04, D08, J11, D11, D15, D16

Short Answers

1. Draw a neat labeled diagram of medial surface of left lung.	232	422	D15(RS3)
2. Root of lung (right)—contents.	233	427	D17(RS3), J98, D15
3. Hilum of right lung (structures present).	233	427	J09(RS2), D98
4. Hilum (root) of left lung.	233	427	D03, J04
5. Blood supply of lungs.	233	433	D09(RS2), J10
6. Draw and label hilum/root of right lung.	234	424	D11, D14
7. Describe the lymphatic drainage of the lungs.	235	434	F21(RS4), D10
8. Differences between right and left principle bronchus and its clinical significance.	235	399	D03
9. Define a bronchopulmonary segment.	238	430	J03
10. Bronchopulmonary segments of left lung (upper lobe).	238	431	J04, J09

Contd...

Contd...

	BDC Vol:1	IBSANT1	
Multiple Choice Questions			
1. False statement regarding broncho-pulmonary segment is: a. Pyramidal in shape b. **It is surrounded by connective tissue** c. Each segment has its own artery d. Each segment drained by its own segmental vein	238	430	J21(RS4)

CHAPTER 26: MEDIASTINUM

Long Essay			
1. Define mediastinum. Mention the contents of posterior mediastinum. Describe the thoracic part of esophagus. Add a note on its applied anatomy.	244, 246, 293	383, 391	D08(RS2)
Short Essays			
1. Division of mediastinum and name the contents of superior mediastinum.	244	386	J11
2. Superior mediastinum—boundaries and contents.	244	387	J09(RS2), J14(RS3), D17(RS3), D08, D14
3. Posterior mediastinum—boundaries and contents.	246	390	D18(RS3), N20(RS3), J99, D03, D07
Short Answers			
1. Superior mediastinum—contents.	244	387	D02, J10, J13
2. Anterior mediastinum—boundaries and contents.	246	390	D11
3. Middle mediastinum—contents.	246	390	J04
4. Posterior mediastinum—contents.	246	391	D07(RS2)

Contd...

ANATOMY

Contd...

	BDC Vol:1	IBSANT1	

CHAPTER 27: PERICARDIUM AND HEART

Long Essays

	BDC Vol:1	IBSANT1	
1. Describe the external features of heart. Describe right atrium under following headings: (a) Borders and surfaces; (b) Relations; (c) External and internal features including openings; (d) Blood supply and nerve supply; (e) Development including that of interatrial septum; (f) Anomalies.	253	440, 445	J06(RS2), D07(RS2), D13(RS3), N20(RS3), D02, D04, J06, D06
2. Describe the external and internal features of the left atrium.	262	445	D13
3. Describe blood supply of heart. Give its applied anatomy. Add a note on development of interatrial septum.	269	460	J11(RS2), D11(RS3), D17(RS3), D19(RS3), D98, D99, D12, J14

Short Essays

	BDC Vol:1	IBSANT1	
1. List the differences in the interior of the right and left atrium.	—	446	J14
2. Pericardium—layers and sinuses.	249	467	J06, D15
3. Fibrous pericardium.	250	467	J03
4. Serous pericardium.	250	469	D10(RS2)
5. Pericardial sinuses.	250	469	D14(RS3), J12
6. Transverse sinus of heart.	250	470	J13(RS3)
7. Oblique sinus of pericardium.	250	469	D13(RS3)
8. Sternocostal surface of heart.	257	442	J98
9. Right atrium.	258	445	D09(RS2), D12(RS3)
10. Describe the interior of the right atrium with a neat labeled diagram.	259	445	J21(RS4), J10(RS2), D07, D16
11. Openings of right atrium.	260	447	J18(RS3)
12. Interatrial septum and its development.	260	448	J05(RS2), D05

Contd...

Contd...

	BDC Vol:1	IBSANT1	
13. Interventricular septum.	261	453	D00
14. Chordae tendinae.	261	450	D17(RS3)
15. Right coronary artery.	269	460	D06(RS2), D12(RS3), D01
16. Left coronary artery.	270	462	D15(RS3), D00
17. Venous drainage of heart.	274	464	J09(RS2), J15(RS3), D09
18. Coronary sinus—formation, course and tributaries.	274	465	J16(RS3), J18(RS3), D98, J01, D03, D10, J11, D11
Short Answers			
1. Triangle of Koch.	—	448	D09
2. Name the layers of the pericardium. Give its nerve supply.	249	467	J21(RS4)
3. Pericardial sinuses.	250	469	D18(RS3)
4. Transverse sinus of pericardium.	250	470	D08(RS2), J02
5. Oblique sinus of pericardium (boundaries).	250	469	J04
6. Openings in right atrium.	258	447	J08(RS2), D98, J05
7. Papillary muscles.	261	450	D01
8. Moderator band.	261	454	D13(RS3), D14(RS3)
9. Where are SA and AV nodes located? Give their blood supply.	269	456	J02
10. Name the branches of right coronary artery.	269	462	D14, D16
11. Areas supplied by right coronary artery.	269	462	J05, J13
12. Branches of left coronary artery and parts of heart supplied.	270	463	J03, J10

Contd...

Contd...

	BDC Vol:1	IBSANT1	
13. Coronary sinus—location, formation, termination, tributaries and development.	274	465	F21(RS4), J05(RS2), J17(RS3), J98
14. Nerve supply of heart (cardiac plexuses).	274	517	D09(RS2), N20(RS3), D01
15. Deep cardiac plexus.	274	512	D15(RS3)

CHAPTER 28: SUPERIOR VENA CAVA, AORTA AND PULMONARY TRUNK

Long Essay

1. Describe arch of aorta under following headings (a) Situation; (b) Origin, course and termination (extent); (c) Relations and branches (including rare branches); (d) Development and anomalies.	281	477	J05, J08

Short Essays

1. Arch of aorta—branches and relations.	281	477	J00, J07, J12, J15
2. Draw and label a cross section of thorax at level of T4.	284	478	D01

Short Answer

1. Arch of aorta—branches.	284	477	D11

CHAPTER 29: TRACHEA, ESOPHAGUS AND THORACIC DUCT

Long Essay

1. Describe thoracic part of esophagus under following headings: (a) Extent; (b) Course and relations; (c) Blood supply and nerve supply; (d) Constrictions, (e) Applied anatomy; (e) Microscopic structure.	292	402	J07, D08

Short Essays

1. Trachea—extent, labeled diagram, applied anatomy.	289	394	J06

Contd...

Contd...

	BDC Vol:1	IBSANT1	
2. Thoracic duct—extent, length, formation, course, relations, area of drainage and termination. Explain how stab injuries to the left side of the neck can damage the thoracic duct.	296	493	F21(RS4), D05(RS2), J07(RS2), J13(RS3), J18(RS3), D19(RS3), J02, D04, D07, J14
Short Answers			
1. Sites of normal constrictions in esophagus and structures compressing it.	293	404	D12(RS3), J03
2. Thoracic duct—commencement and termination.	296	493	D01, J12
Multiple Choice Questions			
1. Surface marking of inferior line of pleural reflection passes through: a. 6th rib along the midaxillary line b. 7th rib along the midaxillary line c. 8th rib along the midaxillary line d. **10th rib along the midaxillary line**	302	414	J21(RS4)

CHAPTER 30: MISCELLANEOUS

Diaphragm though part of Paper I is covered in Abdomen section (please refer it there).

	BDC Vol:2	IBSANT2	
SECTION 4: LOWER LIMB			

CHATER 31: INTRODUCTION

None

CHATER 32: BONES OF LOWER LIMB

Short Essays

1. Ischial tuberosity	13	15	J01
2. Greater trochanter of femur	18	23	J05
3. Patella.	23	30	J13(RS3)
4. Upper end of tibia.	25	32	D00

Contd...

ANATOMY

Contd...

	BDC Vol:2	IBSANT2	
Short Answers			
1. Greater sciatic notch.	8	12	D14(RS3)
2. Ischial spine.	12	15	D05
3. Ischial tuberosity—muscles attached.	13	15	D10, D14
4. Define femoral torsion.	18	—	J99
5. Greater trochanter of femur.	18	23	D05(RS2)
6. Lower end of femur.	19	25	J09
7. Linea aspera of femur.	19	25	J11(RS2)
8. Adductor tubercle.	19	26	J03
9. Muscles attached to femur (greater trochanter/linea aspera).	20	26	J07(RS2), J05, J06
10. Medicolegal importance of ossification center to lower end of femur.	22	—	J01, D04, D07
11. Patella (how it differs from other bones and bursae in relation to it).	23, 151	30	J98, J05
12. How do you differentiate left from right patella?	23	31	D16
13. Tibial tuberosity.	26	32	J04
14. Soleal line.	26	34	D03
15. Structures attached to anterior intercondylar area of tibia.	28	35	D08

CHAPTER 33: FRONT OF THIGH

Long Essays			
1. Describe femoral triangle under following headings: (a) Boundaries; (b) Contents; (c) Applied aspects.	48	136	J13(RS3), D19(RS3), N20(RS3)
2. Describe femoral artery under following headings: (a) Extent (origin and termination); (b) Course and relations; (c) Branches; (d) Anastomoses; (e) Applied anatomy	56	89	J07(RS2), J05
3. Describe femoral nerve under following headings: (a) Origin; (b) Course; (c) Termination; (d) Relations; (e) Branches.	58	66	J03

Contd...

Contd...

	BDC Vol:2	IBSANT2	
Short Essays			
1. Cutaneous nerve supply of front of thigh.	44	86	J14(RS3)
2. Iliotibial tract.	47	134	J18(RS3)
3. A 23-year-old female came to the emergency department with an injury to the middle of the right groin region. On examination, there was a deep lacerated wound just below the middle of the right inguinal ligament. Describe the structures at risk in this region and their relations. Describe the boundaries of the triangle in this region.	48	136	F21(RS4)
4. Femoral triangle—boundaries and contents.	48	136	D10(RS2), D98, D06, D09, J13, J15
5. Femoral sheath—formation, divisions, contents, applied anatomy.	51	138	D05(RS2), D06(RS2), J08(RS2), D09(RS2), D16(RS3), J99, D00, J04, D05, D08, J14
6. Femoral canal (applied anatomy).	51	139	J16(RS3)
7. Profunda femoris artery—origin, course and branches.	57	93	D11(RS3), D18(RS3), J19(RS3), J98, D99, J12
8. Femoral nerve—root value, course, branches.	58	66	J17(RS3), D07, D11
9. Quadriceps femoris.	59	145	J08(RS2)
10. Adductor canal—boundaries and contents.	59	142	J09(RS2), D09(RS2), D15(RS3), D17(RS3), D01, J07, J09, J11, D13

Contd...

Contd...

	BDC Vol:2	IBSANT2	
Short Answers			
1. House maid's knee.	47	245	J18(RS3)
2. Iliotibial tract.	47	134	J15(RS3), D13
3. Saphenous opening.	47	133	J19(RS3)
4. Femoral triangle—boundaries, floor, contents and its posterior relations.	48	136	D99, J01, D04, J07
5. Femoral sheath—formation, division, contents and applied anatomy.	51	138	D08(RS2), J18(RS3), D18(RS3), D04, J07
6. Femoral canal—situation, contents, applied anatomy.	51	139	J17(RS3), D17(RS3), D07, J09, D14
7. Femoral ring.	51	139	J11
8. Branches (superficial) of femoral artery.	57	92	D14(RS3), J08
9. Profunda femoris artery (branches).	57	93	J06(RS2), D15(RS3)
10. Branches of femoral nerve.	59	67	D06(RS2), D09
11. Cutaneous branches of femoral nerve with areas of distribution.	59	68	J98
12. Quadriceps femoris (components and action).	59	145	D13(RS3), J06, D15
13. Sartorius muscle.	61	144	J13(RS3), D08
14. Rectus femoris.	61	145	D14(RS3)
15. Adductor canal—contents.	60	142	D08(RS2), D98
CHAPTER 34: MEDIAL SIDE OF THIGH			
Long Essays			
1. Name the adductor compartment muscles of the thigh (adductors of thigh). Give origin, insertion, morphology, relations, nerve supply, actions and openings and structures passing through the adductor magnus muscle.	62	151	J01, D04

Contd...

Contd...

	BDC Vol:2	IBSANT2	
2. Describe the: (a) Formation; (b) Course; (c) Branches and; (d) Applied anatomy of obturator nerve.	65	65	J15
Short Essays			
1. Adductor magnus muscle.	63	151	D06(RS2), D19(RS3), D03
2. Obturator nerve—root value, course, branches, applied anatomy.	65	65	D08
Short Answers			
1. Adductor muscles.	63	151	D07(RS2)
2. Nerve supply to adductor muscles.	63	151	J11
3. Adductor longus.	63	151	J14(RS3)
4. Pectineus.	63	151	D05(RS2)
5. Two functional components of Adductor magnus.	63	151	J99
6. The obturator nerve was injured in an anterior dislocation of hip joint. All the muscles supplied by this nerve were paralysed except part of one muscle. Which muscle is this and what is the anatomical basis? Enumerate the muscles supplied by the obturator nerve.	63, 66	151, 65	F21(RS4)
7. Obturator nerve—root value, muscles supplied.	65	65	J05(RS2), J07
8. Structure supplied by anterior division of obturator nerve.	66	65	D99
CHAPTER 35: GLUTEAL REGION			
Long Essays			
1. Enumerate structures under cover of Gluteus maximus. Describe in detail Sciatic nerve and its applied anatomy.	74, 90	168, 72	D17(RS3)
2. Describe the gluteus maximus muscle under the following headings: origin, insertion, nerve supply and action. Add a note on structures under cover of gluteus maximus.	72, 74	163, 168	J16(RS3)

Contd...

ANATOMY

Contd...

	BDC Vol:2	IBSANT2	
3. A 14-year-old boy came with altered gait a few hours after an injection in his right buttock. On clinical examination he was found to be having right foot drop. a. What is the anatomical basis for the boy's symptoms? b. Describe the following structures under the cover of the gluteus maximus muscle (i) Vessels, (ii) Nerves.	85, 74	74, 168	F21(RS4)
Short Essays			
1. Gluteus maximus muscle—origin, insertion, nerve supply and actions.	72	163	J19(RS3), J05, D08
2. Gluteus medius and minimus.	72	163	J10(RS2)
3. Piriformis muscle.	72	164	D14(RS3), D98
4. Greater sciatic foramen.	78	17	D02
5. Lesser sciatic foramen—formation and structures transmitted.	78	17	J10
Short Answers			
1. Name glutei muscle and their nerve supply.	72	163	D06(RS2)
2. Gluteus maximus muscle (Insertion, any two actions).	72	163	J21(RS4), J08(RS2)
3. Gamelli muscles.	72	164	J11
4. Obturator internus—nerve supply and action.	72	164	J15(RS3)
5. Draw a neat labeled diagram of structures undercover of gluteus maximus.	73	168	J13(RS3)
6. Name muscles supplied by superior gluteal nerve and mention their actions.	76	70	J98, D12
7. Inferior gluteal nerve.	76	70	J14(RS3)
8. Cruciate anastomosis—formation and applied aspect.	78	99	J05(RS2), J15(RS3), J18(RS3), N20(RS3), J99, J10

Contd...

Contd...

	BDC Vol:2	IBSANT2	
9. Structures passing through greater sciatic foramen.	78	17	J05(RS2)
10. Name the structures emerging above and below the piriformis muscle.	78	17	J13, D15

CHAPTER 36: POPLITEAL FOSSA

Long Essay

1. Describe popliteal fossa under following headings: (a) Boundaries; (b) Contents; (c) Applied anatomy; Describe origin, course and branches of popliteal artery.	80	177	D05(RS2), D12(RS3), D01, D07, J12

Short Essays

1. Popliteal fossa—boundaries and contents.	80	177	D08(RS2), J05, D12, D14
2. Popliteal artery—origin, termination and branches.	82	99	D05, D11
3. Common peroneal (lateral popliteal) nerve—origin, course and branches.	84	80	D15(RS3), D05, J13, D15

Short Answers

1. Popliteal fossa—boundaries and contents.	80	177	D17(RS3), D04
2. Popliteal artery—branches.	82	99	D09
3. Foot drop.	85	81	D07(RS2), J01, D04

CHAPTER 37: BACK OF THIGH

Long Essays

1. Name hamstrings of thigh. Mention origin, insertion, nerve supply and actions of semimembranosus.	87	172	J06
2. Describe sciatic nerve under following headings: (a) Root value; (b) Origin; (c) Course and relations; (d) Branches; (e) Applied anatomy.	90	72	J05(RS2), D10(RS2), D11(RS3), J02, D09, D10

Contd...

ANATOMY

Contd...

	BDC Vol:2	IBSANT2	
Short Essays			
1. Hamstring muscles.	87	172	D07(RS2), J11(RS2), N20(RS3)
2. Biceps femoris muscle.	89	174	J17(RS3), D99
3. Sciatic nerve—relations and branches of distribution.	90	72	J15(RS3)
Short Answers			
1. Hamstring muscles—enumerate, nerve supply and characteristic features.	87	172	J10, D13
2. Semimembranosus muscle	89	174	D12(RS3)

CHAPTER 38: FRONT, LATERAL AND MEDIAL SIDES OF LEG AND DORSUM OF FOOT

Long Essay			
1. Name dorsiflexors of ankle joint. Describe the origin, insertion, nerve supply and actions of the dorsiflexors of the ankle joint (extensor digitorum longus). Explain the anatomical basis of foot drop.	99, 101	184, 168	J21(RS4), J07
Short Essays			
1. Cutaneous nerve supply of dorsum of foot.	94	181	D13(RS3), D14(RS3), D16
2. Retinaculae around ankle joint.	95	188	J11, J15
3. Extensor retinaculum of foot.	96	189	J05(RS2), D07(RS2), D11(RS3)
4. Interosseous membrane of leg—Muscles attached.	99	—	J07
5. Deep peroneal nerve.	101	83	D09(RS2)
6. Dorsalis pedis artery—formation, termination, relations and branches.	102	106	D05(RS2), J06(RS2), J08(RS2), D17(RS3), N20(RS3)
7. Superficial peroneal nerve.	105	81	D99

Contd...

Contd...

	BDC Vol:2	IBSANT2	
Short Answers			
1. Great saphenous nerve—origin, course and distribution.	94	68	J19(RS3), J05
2. Sensory nerve supply of dorsum of foot.	94	181	J11(RS2), J19(RS3), J05, D11
3. Name the structures passing under the extensor retinaculum of foot.	96	191	D15
4. Tibialis anterior.	99	185	J10
5. Muscles supplied by deep peroneal nerve (anterior tibial nerve).	101	83	J02, J08, J14
6. Dorsalis pedis artery (origin and branches).	102	106	D06(RS2), J13(RS3), J05, D13
7. Peroneus longus muscle.	105	193	J10(RS2), J16(RS3), D09
8. Superficial peroneal nerve—muscles supplied.	104	81	D14(RS3)
9. Anserine bursa.	106	—	D08(RS2)
CHAPTER 39: BACK OF LEG			
Short Essays			
1. Flexor retinaculum of foot—attachments, structures passing underneath.	109	202	J02, D04, J06, J10, J12
2. Explain the attachments, action and nerve supply of the triceps surae muscle.	111	200	J13
3. Popliteus—attachments, nerve supply, action.	113	206	J06(RS2), D10(RS2), D13(RS3), J98, D02, J04, J06
4. Peroneal artery.	117	106	J03
5. Tibial nerve.	117	74	J12(RS3)
Short Answers			
1. Sural nerve (area supplied).	108	75	D13(RS3), J06

Contd...

Contd...

	BDC Vol:2	IBSANT2	
2. Structures passing deep to flexor retinaculum of foot.	109	202	D00, J14
3. Tendocalcaneus.	112	200	J05(RS2), D09(RS2), J10(RS2)
4. Peripheral heart.	112	210	J18(RS3)
5. Popliteus muscle—attachments, action and nerve supply.	113	206	J09(RS2), J09

CHAPTER 40: SOLE OF FOOT

Short Essays

1. Plantar aponeurosis.	120	213	D02
2. Dorsal interossei muscles of sole.	126	222	D10
3. Plantar (arterial) arch.	129	109	J05, D06

Short Answers

1. Name the muscles supplied by the medial plantar nerve in the sole.	128	76	D16
2. Mention the muscles supplied by the lateral plantar nerve.	129	78	J13

CHAPTER 41: VENOUS AND LYMPHATIC DRAINAGE; COMPARISON OF LOWER AND UPPER LIMBS

Long Essay

1. Describe the venous drainage of lower limb with its applied importance.	131	112	J14(RS3)

Short Essays

1. Great saphenous vein/long saphenous vein—origin, course, tributaries and termination.	132	113	J12(RS3), D13(RS3), N20(RS3), D02, D03, J10, D14, D16
2. Small saphenous vein—formation, course, tributaries.	133	115	D08
3. Varicose veins in lower limb.	134	120	J08

Contd...

Contd...

	BDC Vol:2	IBSANT2	
4. Inguinal lymph nodes (superficial)—groups, location, area of drainage and applied importance.	135	123	J21(RS4), J00, D00, D07
Short Answers			
1. Great saphenous vein (origin, termination, named tributaries).	132	113	J06(RS2), D01, D12
2. Veins connected by medial ankle perforators.	134	119	D11(RS3)
3. Varicose veins.	134	120	J09(RS2), J99
4. Inguinal lymph nodes (superficial group).	135	123	J06(RS2), D19(RS3), J09
5. Areas of drainage of horizontal superficial inguinal lymph nodes.	135	125	J01, D04
6. Areas of drainage of popliteal lymph nodes.	136	124	J07

CHAPTER 42: JOINTS OF LOWER LIMB

Long Essays

1. Describe hip joint under following headings: (a) Type and bones taking part (formation/articular surfaces); (b) Capsule and ligaments; (c) Relations;(d) Movements and muscles producing them; (e) Neurovascular supply; (f) Applied anatomy.	140	229	J12(RS3), J06(RS2), D09(RS2), J17(RS3), J19(RS3), J04, J08, J10, J14, D16
2. Describe knee joint under following headings: (a) Type and Bones articulating; (b) Capsule and ligaments; (c) Intraarticular structures (menisci and cruciate ligaments); (d) Blood supply and nerve supply; (e) Movements and muscles producing them; (f) Locking and unlocking movements; (g) Bursae around knee joint; (h) Applied anatomy.	146	236	J08(RS2), J18(RS3), D03, D06, D12

Contd...

Contd...

	BDC Vol:2	IBSANT2	
3. Describe intracapsular structures of knee joint. Add a note on locking and unlocking of knee joint.	149, 153	239, 247	J09(RS2)
4. Describe ankle joint under following headings: (a) Type; (b) Capsule and ligaments; (c) Relations; (d) Movements and muscles producing them; (e) Blood supply; (f) Applied anatomy.	155	249	J10(RS2), J00, D11
5. Describe inversion and eversion. Name joints in which these movements occur and name muscles producing these movements, with their attachments and nerve supply in a tabulated form.	161	253	J09
Short Essays			
1. Describe the articular surfaces and movements of the hip joint.	140	229	D15
2. Ligaments of hip joint.	140	230	D15(RS3)
3. Iliofemoral ligament—attachments and applied anatomy.	141	232	J05(RS2), J06
4. Abductors of hip joint.	144	235	D16(RS3)
5. Medial ligaments of knee (tibial collateral ligament).	148	239	J02
6. Intra-articular structures of knee joint.	149	239	J15
7. Lateral ligaments of knee.	149	240	D04
8. Cruciate ligaments of knee joint.	149	241	D08(RS2), J17(RS3), D01
9. Semilunar cartilage (medial meniscus).	150	241	D99, D14
10. Movements of knee joint.	152	246	J11
11. Locking and unlocking movements of knee joint.	149	247	D05(RS2), D14(RS3)
12. Deltoid ligament of ankle joint.	156	250	J07(RS2), J09(RS2), J07

Contd...

Contd...

	BDC Vol:2	IBSANT2	
13. Movements and applied anatomy of ankle joint.	156	251	J08
14. Tibiofibular joints.	158	248	D18(RS3)
15. Spring ligament.	160	253	J01
16. Inversion and eversion of foot—joints involved and muscles acting.	161	253	D06(RS2), J16(RS3), D05, D09, D14
Short Answers			
1. Iliofemoral ligament.	141	232	D07(RS2), D14
2. Muscles performing lateral rotation of thigh (lateral rotator muscles of the hip joint).	144	235	D10(RS2)
3. Abductors of hip joint.	144	235	J06
4. Name the ligaments of the knee joint.	146	239	D13
5. Capsule of knee joint.	146	238	J13(RS3)
6. Ligamentum patellae (patellar ligament).	148	240	D11(RS3), J16(RS3), D13
7. Tibial collateral (medial) ligament of knee joint.	148	239	J08(RS2), J05
8. Enumerate intra-articular structures in knee joint.	149	239	J10
9. Cruciate ligaments.	149	241	D17(RS3)
10. Medial meniscus.	150	242	D16(RS3)
11. Functions of menisci of knee joint.	150	241	D09
12. Bursa around knee joint.	151	244	D12(RS3)
13. Mention the genicular nerves supplying the knee joint.	151	246	J13
14. Muscles causing medial rotations of knee joint.	152	247	J07
15. Locking and unlocking of knee joint.	152	247	J17(RS3)
16. What is meant by locking of knee joint?	152	247	D11

Contd...

ANATOMY

Contd...

	BDC Vol:2	IBSANT2	
17. Deltoid ligament—attachments.	156	250	J98, J10
18. Name subtaloid joints and mention movements possible in it.	159	252	J98
19. Spring ligament—attachments.	160	253	D16(RS3), J99
20. Define eversion of foot. Muscles responsible for eversion of foot (evertors of foot) and their nerve supply.	161	253	D16(RS3), D99

Multiple Choice Questions

1. The unlocking of knee joint is done by _____ muscle:
   a. Vastus lateralis
   b. Vastus medialis
   c. Biceps femoris
   d. **Popliteus**

CHAPTER 43: ARCHES OF FOOT

Long Essay

1. Name and describe arches of foot (lateral longitudinal/medial longitudinal) under the following heads. (a) Types and bones taking part; (b) Factors maintaining the arches and; (c) Applied aspect.	164	254	D07(RS2), D08(RS2), J15(RS3), D15(RS3), D16(RS3), D18(RS3), D98, D00

Short Essay

1. Longitudinal arches of foot (medial longitudinal arch of foot).	164	254	D10(RS2), J16(RS3), J99, J03, J09, D13

Short Answers

1. Medial longitudinal arch of foot.	164	254	J11(RS2)
2. Bones forming medial longitudinal arch of foot.	164	254	D06(RS2), J07(RS2), D15
3. Bones forming lateral longitudinal arch of foot.	165	255	D09(RS2), D08

Contd...

Contd...

	BDC Vol:2	IBSANT2	
CHAPTER 44: MISCELLANEOUS			
Multiple Choice Question			
1. In the radiograph of hip joint the normal relation of the head of femur with acetabulum is indicated by _______. a. Hilton's line b. **Shenton's line** c. Holden's line d.. Nelaton's line	145	235	J21(RS4)
SECTION 5: ABDOMEN AND PELVIS			
CHAPTER 45: INTRODUCTION TO ABDOMEN AND OSTEOLOGY			
Short Essay			
1. Compare and contrast the features of the male and female bony pelvis.	199	285	F21(RS4)
Short Answers			
1. Structure related to pelvic surface of sacrum.	—	—	D05(RS2)
2. Sacral hiatus.	194	281	D13(RS3)
3. Sacral canal (contents).	194	—	J14(RS3), D00
4. Differences between male and female bony pelvis.	199	285	J16(RS3)
CHAPTER 46: ANTERIOR ABDOMINAL WALL			
Long Essays			
1. Describe rectus sheath under following headings: (a) Formation at different levels; (b) Contents; (c) Applied anatomy.	214	305	D12(RS3), D16(RS3), D02, D13
2. Describe inguinal canal under following headings: (a) Location and extent; (b) Openings; (c) Boundaries; (d) Contents (structures passing through); (e) Natural safety mechanisms (factors preventing inguinal hernias); (f) Applied anatomy. Add a note on inguinal hernias.	216	297	D05(RS2), J10(RS2), J13(RS3), D17(RS3), J02, D03, J09, J15, D15

Contd...

Contd...

	BDC Vol:2	IBSANT2	
Short Essays			
1. Transpyloric plane.	201	—	D13(RS3)
2. Umbilicus.	202	290	J16(RS3), J00
3. Anterior abdominal wall—blood supply and nerve supply.	203	308	J03
4. External oblique muscle.	207	299	J01
5. Rectus abdominis.	209	304	D01
6. Inguinal ligament—attachment and expansions.	211	294	J11(RS2), J19(RS3)
7. Conjoint tendon.	211	296	D00
8. Rectus sheath—formation, contents and applied anatomy.	214	305	D10(RS2), D14(RS3), J04, D09, D10
9. Inguinal canal—boundaries and contents; Defensive mechanism.	216	297	J17(RS3), J11
10. Spermatic cord—coverings, contents.	218	300	J10(RS2), J00, D01, J04, J09
11. Protective mechanism of inguinal canal.	218	302	D12(RS3)
12. Inguinal hernia—types, coverings	219	303	D07
13. Indirect inguinal hernia.	220	303	D10
Short Answers			
1. Physiological umbilical hernia.	—	291	J04
2. Hesselbach's triangle.	—	303	D12(RS3)
3. Transpyloric plane and structures lie on it.	201	—	J07(RS2), J16(RS3), D16(RS3), J18(RS3), J98
4. Raspberry tumor.	203	—	J05
5. Ilioinguinal nerve.	205	308	J16(RS3), J09
6. Inguinal ligament.	211	294	J05
7. Cremasteric reflex.	211	—	J10

Contd...

Contd...

	BDC Vol:2	IBSANT2	
8. Conjoint tendon.	211	296	J15(RS3)
9. Cremaster.	211	302	J16(RS3)
10. Pyramidalis muscle—attachments.	212	305	D13(RS3), J14(RS3), D15(RS3), J15
11. Rectus sheath—muscles forming, contents.	214	305	D18(RS3), D19(RS3), J05, J10
12. Mention the layers present in the anterior wall of the rectus sheath at different levels.	214	306	D12
13. Inguinal rings (superficial/deep).	216	300	D07(RS2), D08, D10, D14
14. Mention the contents of the inguinal canal.	218	300	D14(RS3), D11
15. Spermatic cord—coverings, contents.	218	300	D07(RS2), J15(RS3), J17(RS3), D99, D07, J08
16. Name the coverings of the spermatic cord, and what are they derived from?	218	301	J14
17. Name the structures protecting the superficial and deep inguinal ring.	218	300	D12
18. Sites of hernia in the abdomen.	219	—	D99
19. What is indirect inguinal hernia?	220	303	J13
20. List the differences between direct and indirect inguinal hernia.	222	—	D13
Multiple Choice Questions			
1. Superficial inguinal ring is a triangular gap in ________. a. Superficial fascia b. **External oblique aponeurosis** c. Internal oblique aponeurosis d. Fascia transversalis	216	300	J21(RS4)

Contd...

Contd...

	BDC Vol:2	IBSANT2	
CHAPTER 47: MALE EXTERNAL GENITAL ORGANS			
Long Essays			
1. Describe testis under following headings: (a) Location and gross features; (b) Blood supply; (c) Lymphatic drainage; (d) Development.	229	319	J06
2. Describe the coverings, microstructure (diagrammatic) and development of testis.	230, 232	320	D14(RS3)
Short Essays			
1. Thermoregulation of testis.	—	—	D16(RS3)
2. Ectopic testis.	233	322	J10(RS2)
3. Descent of testis.	233	322	J18(RS3), D02, D05, J08, D12
Short Answers			
1. Contents in the body of the penis.	224	316	D13
2. Name the layers present in the scrotum.	228	315	D15
3. Testis—labeled diagram.	229	320	J07
4. Coverings (tunicae) of testis.	230	320	D06(RS2), D19(RS3), D07
5. What is tunica vaginalis? And what is the congenital anomaly associated with it?	230	320	D16
6. Venous drainage of testis (testicular vein).	231	322	J21(RS4), J08(RS2)
7. Pampiniform plexus of veins.	231	322	D15(RS3)
8. Lymphatic drainage of testis.	231	322	D14
9. Mention the congenital anomalies associated with descent of the testis.	233	322	J13
10. What are the anatomical reasons for the left testicular varicosity?	233	322	D13

Contd...

Contd...

	BDC Vol:2	IBSANT2	
11. Descent of testis (factors involved).	233	322	D08(RS2), D12(RS3), D99, D09
12. Gubernaculum testis.	233	—	N20(RS3), D01, J03

CHPATER 48: ABDOMINAL CAVITY AND PERITONEUM

Short Essays

1. Greater omentum—attachments, contents and functions.	241	346	D12(RS3), J14(RS3), J03, D07
2. Lesser omentum—attachments, contents.	243	345	D11(RS3), D16(RS3), D18(RS3), D01, J04, D05, J07, D08
3. Mesentery of small intestine—attachments and contents.	244	352	J07(RS2), D14(RS3), J16(RS3), D18(RS3), J99, J02, D04, J09, D09, J13
4. Describe the vertical disposition of the peritoneum.	246	341	D13
5. Epiploic foramen.	249	344	D06(RS2), D10(RS2), J13(RS3), J00, J02, D03, D04
6. Lesser sac (omental bursa)—location, boundaries, openings, applied anatomy.	248	347	J05(RS2), D07(RS2), J11(RS2), D17(RS3), D98, J01, J05, J07, J08, J09, D16
7. Hepatorenal pouch.	250	349	D06(RS2), D08(RS2)

Contd...

Contd...

	BDC Vol:2	IBSANT2	
8. Rectouterine pouch (Pouch of Douglas).	250	342	D13(RS3), J17(RS3), J10
9. Peritoneal recesses	252	348	D10
Short Answers			
1. Ileocecal folds.	—	—	J09(RS2)
2. Ovarian bursa.	—	—	J09(RS2)
3. Lesser omentum (contents).	243	345	N20(RS3), J06, J10
4. Mesentery—attachments, borders and contents.	244	352	J17(RS3), J01
5. Root of mesentery—attachments and contents.	244	352	J19(RS3), J12
6. List the structures crossed by the root of the mesentery.	244	352	D12, D13
7. Structures attached to the root of the transverse mesocolon.	245	352	J14
8. Name the contents of the transverse mesocolon.	245	352	D11
9. Sigmoid mesocolon.	245	353	D14
10. Name the peritoneal ligaments/folds attached to the liver.	246	341	D13
11. Name the umbilical fold and mention their contents.	248	341	J14
12. Epiploic foramen (draw and label/ boundaries).	249	344	D05(RS2), J06(RS2), D07(RS2), J10(RS2), J18(RS3), D19(RS3), J98, J08, J12, D12, J15
13. Omental bursa.	249	347	J08(RS2)
14. Morrison's hepatorenal pouch.	251	349	D18(RS3)
15. Rectouterine pouch (Douglas pouch)—parts, clinical importance.	251	342	J05(RS2), J12(RS3), J15

Contd...

Contd...

	BDC Vol:2	IBSANT2	
16. Name the paraduodenal recesses and mention its applied importance.	252	351	J13
17. Peritoneal recesses in relation to cecum and appendix.	252	351	J99
Multiple Choice Questions			
1. The epiploic foramen is bounded superiorly by ___________. a. **Caudate process of liver** b. First part of duodenum c. Right free margin of lesser omentum d. Inferior vena cava	249	345	J21(RS4)

CHAPTER 49: ABDOMINAL PART OF ESOPHAGUS AND STOMACH

Long Essay			
1. Describe stomach under following headings: (a) Position; (b) Parts; (c) Gross features; (d) Peritoneal and visceral relations; (e) Blood supply and venous drainage; (f) Nerve supply; (g) Lymphatic drainage; (h) Development and congenital anomalies; (i) Microscopic structure; (j) Applied anatomy.	257	359	J07(RS2), J14(RS3), J99, D00, J05, D06, D08, D09, D11, J13, D13, D14
Short Essays			
1. Describe the parts and blood supply/lymphatic drainage of the stomach.	257	359	D19(RS3), D16
2. Stomach bed.	258	361	J06(RS2), J15(RS3), J16(RS3), D02
3. Blood supply and lymphatic drainage of stomach.	260	363	J12(RS3)
4. Stomach—blood supply.	260	363	J08(RS2), D10(RS2), D14(RS3), N20(RS3)
5. Stomach—lymphatic drainage.	260	364	D08(RS2), D09(RS2), D03

Contd...

Contd...

	BDC Vol:2	IBSANT2	
Short Answers			
1. Name the types of stomach.	—	—	D12
2. Fundus of stomach.	260	359	J15
3. Name the peritoneal folds attached to the stomach.	260	363	D15
4. Structures in stomach bed.	260	361	D99, J08, J10, D10
5. A patient is brought to the emergency department with a history of a stab wound to the abdomen. The structures forming the stomach bed are injured. Name any six structures forming the stomach bed.	260	361	J21(RS4)
6. Blood supply of stomach.	260	363	D16(RS3), D18(RS3)
7. Lymphatic drainage of stomach.	260	364	F21(RS4), J11(RS2

CHAPTER 50: SMALL AND LARGE INTESTINES

Long Essays			
1. Describe the duodenum under the following headings: (a) Position and parts; (b) Peritoneal and visceral relations; (c) Blood supply; (d) Development.	268	368	D16
2. Describe 2nd part of duodenum under following headings: (a) Relations; (b) Internal features; (c) Arterial supply; (d) Development; (e) Applied anatomy.	270	368	D99
Short Essays			
1. Describe the parts, peritoneal attachments and blood supply of the duodenum.	268	368	D13, D15
2. Second part of the duodenum—extent, relations, blood supply and development.	270	368	J06(RS2), J12(RS3), J15(RS3), J18(RS3), J19(RS3), J04, D06

Contd...

Contd...

	BDC Vol:2	IBSANT2	
3. Meckel's diverticulum.	275	378	D05(RS2), J13(RS3)
4. Blood supply of colon (large intestine).	278	401	J13(RS3), J00
5. Cecum (parts, position and blood supply).	280	392	D06(RS2), D11(RS3), J13(RS3), D19(RS3), J12, J13
6. Vermiform appendix—situation, positions, peritoneal relations, blood supply, microscopic structure and applied anatomy.	283	395	J06(RS2), D10(RS2), D12(RS3), J98, D99, J08, D08, J11, J14
7. A 26-year-old male presented to the emergency department with complaints of pain in the umbilical region which later shifted to the right iliac fossa. There was tenderness elicited at McBurney's point. A clinical diagnosis of acute appendicitis was made. a. Explain the anatomical basis of the pain that was initially felt in the umbilical region. b. Explain why the pain later shifted to the right iliac fossa? c. What is McBurney's point and its clinical importance? d. Describe the positions of the appendix. e. Describe the arterial supply of the appendix.	284	398	F21(RS4)
Short Answers			
1. Interior of second part of duodenum.	270	369	F21(RS4), J12
2. Suspensory ligament of duodenum/ Ligament of Treitz.	272	374	J14(RS3), D14(RS3), D00, J01, D04, J15

Contd...

ANATOMY

Contd...

	BDC Vol:2	IBSANT2	
3. What is suspensory ligament of the duodenum and what does it represent embryologically?	272	374	J14
4. Blood supply of 2nd part of duodenum.	272	374	J09
5. Duodenal cap.	274	376	D00
6. Differences between jejunum and ileum—gross and microscopic.	275	377	J19(RS3)
7. Meckel's diverticulum—embryological basis.	275	378	F21(RS4), D12(RS3), D16(RS3), D01, D03, D10
8. Parts of large intestine.	277	391	J06(RS2)
9. *Taenia coli.*	277	392	J00, D00
10. Appendices epiploicae.	277	392	J09
11. Difference between large intestine and small intestine.	279	392	D12(RS3), D16
12. Types of cecum.	281	393	J10
13. Name the features in the interior of the cecum.	281	394	D16
14. Ileocecal valve.	281	394	D18(RS3)
15. Vermiform appendix—positions (normal and abnormal).	283	395	J07(RS2), J15(RS3), D17(RS3), J19(RS3), D00, D04, D11, D15
16. Mc Burney's point and its applied importance.	284	398	J08(RS2), J15(RS3), J01, D02, D04, J09, D09
17. Transverse colon.	285	400	J19(RS3)
18. Sigmoid colon.	286	400	D12(RS3)

Contd...

Contd...

	BDC Vol:2	IBSANT2	
CHAPTER 51: LARGE BLOOD VESSELS OF THE GUT			
Long Essay			
1. Describe portal vein under following headings: (a) Formation; (b) Termination; (c) Course and Tributaries; (d) Portocaval anastomosis with systemic veins; (e) Development; (f) Applied anatomy.	292	473	J15(RS3), D98, D01
Short Essays			
1. Celiac trunk (relations, branches and viscera supplied).	287	458	J08(RS2), D12(RS3), D98, J99, J03, J08, J12, D12
2. Right gastric artery—course, branches and area of distribution.	288	462	J21(RS4)
3. Superior mesenteric artery—origin, course and branches.	289	463	J05(RS2), J14(RS3), J19(RS3), D03
4. Inferior mesenteric artery.	290	467	D13(RS3), D02, J05, D11
5. Portal vein—formation, course, relations, tributaries and termination.	292	473	J09(RS2), D09(RS2), J12(RS3), J14
6. Portocaval anastomoses—sites and applied anatomy.	294	476	J07(RS2), D07(RS2), J11(RS2), J14(RS3), D17(RS3), J18(RS3), J00, D02, J08, J15
Short Answers			
1. Celiac trunk—branches.	288	458	D08(RS2), D10, D16
2. Splenic artery.	289	463	J16(RS3)
3. Superior mesenteric artery—branches.	289	463	J13, D15

Contd...

ANATOMY

Contd...

	BDC Vol:2	IBSANT2	
4. Arteries supplying transverse colon.	291	468	J05
5. Inferior mesenteric artery—branches.	291	467	D09(RS2)
6. Name the structures supplied by the inferior mesenteric artery.	291	467	D12
7. Marginal artery of Drummond.	291	468	J10
8. How is the marginal artery of the colon formed?	291	468	J14
9. Sites of portosystemic anastomoses.	294	476	J06(RS2), J99, D11
10. What is the clinical significance of portocaval anastomosis?	294	476	D15
11. Caput medusae.	294	476	D00
Multiple Choice Questions			
1. Following all arteries are branches of celiac trunk, *except*: a. **Superior mesenteric** b. Left gastric c. Common hepatic d. Splenic	289	458	J21(RS4)
CHAPTER 52: EXTRAHEPATIC BILIARY APPARATUS			
Long Essays			
1. Draw a neat labeled diagram to show the components of the extrahepatic biliary system. Describe the gallbladder under the following headings: (a) Location; (b) Parts; (c) Relations; (d) Blood supply; and (e) Applied anatomy.	297	419	F21(RS4)
2. Describe the extrahepatic biliary apparatus.	297	419	J12(RS3)
Short Essays			
1. Gallbladder.	297	420	J98, D98, D99, D01, D11
2. Bile duct (formation, termination and relations).	299	420	J11(RS2), D11(RS3), J00, J01, J03, D05

Contd...

Contd...

	BDC Vol:2	IBSANT2	
Short Answers			
1. Structures forming extrahepatic biliary apparatus.	297	419	J06
2. What are the parts of the gallbladder?	298	420	J13, D15
3. Location of fundus of gallbladder.	298	420	J07
4. Ampula of Vater.	300	420	J11
5. Sphincters related to bile and pancreatic duct.	300	422	J08
6. Calot's triangle—boundaries and contents.	300	423	J21(RS4)

CHAPTER 53: SPLEEN, PANCREAS AND LIVER

Long Essays			
1. Describe spleen under following headings: (a) Situation, size and shape; (b) Borders and surfaces; (c) Peritoneal and visceral relations; (d) Ligaments; (e) Blood supply; (f) Development; (g) Microscopic structure; (h) Functions; (i) Applied anatomy.	305	385	D07, J08
2. Describe pancreas under following headings: (a) Position; (b) Gross features (parts); (c) Peritoneal and visceral relations; (d) Ducts; (e) Blood supply; (f) Lymphatic drainage; (g) Development; (h) Microscopic anatomy; (i) Applied anatomy.	310	380	D06(RS2), J11(RS2), D15(RS3), J04, J11, D12
3. Describe gross anatomy of head of pancreas under the following headings: (a) Situation and gross features; (b) Relations; (c) Blood supply; (d) Development.	310	380	D10(RS2), J98
4. Describe the gross anatomy of Liver with its applied aspects.	318	406	D14(RS3)
Short Essays			
1. Spleen—situation, surfaces (visceral), relations, blood supply.	305	3385	D09(RS2), J02, D04, D05, D06, J09

Contd...

ANATOMY

Contd...

	BDC Vol:2	IBSANT2	
2. Ligaments of spleen—attachments, contents and development.	307	387	J06(RS2), J09(RS2), J04
3. Ligaments and relations of spleen.	307	386	J15(RS3)
4. Hilum of the spleen—contents.	308	386	J06
5. Head of pancreas—relations and blood supply.	310	380	J21(RS4), J10(RS2), J12
6. Relations of pancreas.	312	382	D10
7. Blood supply and development of pancreas.	315	384	D14
8. Porta hepatis—location, contents and applied anatomy.	320	411	J06, J09
9. Ligaments of liver.	321	413	J19(RS3)
10. Inferior surface of liver.	322	411	D06
Short Answers			
1. Ligaments (peritoneal) of spleen—attachments, contents.	322	387	D06(RS2), D10(RS2), D16(RS3), J98, D99, J12, D16
2. Lienorenal ligament.	307	387	J19(RS3)
3. Spleen—relations.	307	386	N20(RS3)
4. Visceral surface of spleen (relations, impressions).	307	386	J01, J07, D08, D15
5. Splenic circulation.	307	389	J13(RS3)
6. Name the parts and secretions of the pancreas.	310	380	D13
7. Uncinate process of pancreas.	312	380	J15
8. Porta hepatis.	320	411	J06(RS2), D05
9. Ligaments (supports) of liver.	321	413	D10
10. Name the lobes of liver.	320	412	J15
11. Anatomical and physiological lobes of liver.	320	412	D99

Contd...

Contd...

	BDC Vol:2	IBSANT2	
12. Bare areas of liver (boundaries).	321	413	J07(RS2), J08(RS2), D18(RS3), N20(RS3), J99, J01, D04, J07, J08, D11, D14
13. Boundaries of bare area of liver.	321	411	D11
14. What are the embryological remnants associated with the liver?	321	417	D16
15. Segments of liver.	324	412	J13(RS3)

CHAPTER 54: KIDNEY AND URETER

Long Essays

1. Describe kidneys (right and left) under following headings: (a) Location, size, borders and surfaces (general features); (b) Coverings; (c) Relations (visceral and peritoneal); (d) Blood supply; (e) Development and congenital anomalies; (f) Applied anatomy	328	429	D07(RS2), D05, J07, J10, J12, J14
2. Describe the coverings, micro-structure (diagram only) and development of kidney.	329	434	D13(RS3)

Short Essays

1. Relations of right kidney.	330	431	J07(RS2), J03, D14
2. Relations of left kidney.	330	431	J15
3. Anterior relations of (right/left) kidney.	330	431	J08(RS2), D19(RS3)
4. Coverings of kidney.	330	434	J98, D03
5. Renal fascia.	330	434	J01
6. Vascular segments of kidney.	336	437	D08
7. Ureter—formation, course, relations (abdominal parts), arterial supply and constrictions.	339	441	F21(RS4), J14(RS3), J15(RS3), J18(RS3), D12

Contd...

Contd...

	BDC Vol:2	IBSANT2	
8. Left ureter (in females).	339	441	J02
9. Right ureter (in females).	339	441	D00, D04, D09
Short Answers			
1. Posterior relations of kidney.	330	431	J05
2. Posterior relations of left kidney.	330	431	D15(RS3), D13
3. Muscles related to posterior surface of right kidney.	330	431	D99
4. Relations of anterior surface of right kidney.	330	431	D10(RS2)
5. Anterior relations of left kidney.	330	431	D09
6. Coverings of kidney.	330	434	J07, D10, J13
7. Labeled diagram of anterior surface of right kidney.	331	432	D00
8. Segments of kidney.	336	437	J15(RS3)
9. Constrictions of ureter—sites/bony landmarks.	340	444	J19(RS3), J11, D11, J12, D13
10. Pelvic part of ureter.	340	441	J12(RS3)

CHAPTER 55: SUPRARENAL GLAND AND CHROMAFFIN SYSTEM

Long Essay			
1. Describe suprarenal glands under following headings: (a) Location and gross features; (b) Relations; (c) Blood supply; (d) Development.	346	446	J01, D04
Short Essay			
1. Suprarenal glands (right/left)—position, coverings, relations, blood supply, development, applied anatomy.	346	446	D05(RS2), J11(RS2), D18(RS3), D98, J05, J06, J07, D08, D15
Short Answers			
1. Layers of suprarenal cortex and hormones secreted by each layer.	348	447	D09(RS2)

Contd...

Contd...

	BDC Vol:2	IBSANT2	
2. Blood supply of suprarenal gland (arterial supply and venous drainage).	348	449	J06(RS2), J09(RS2), D19(RS3), J09, J12, J13

CHAPTER 56: DIAPHRAGM

Long Essay			
1. Describe the thoracoabdominal diaphragm under following headings: (a) Attachments; (b) Openings and structures passing through; (c) Actions and nerve supply; (d) Applied anatomy; (e) Congenital anomalies.	351	361	J16(RS3), J18(RS3), J13
Short Essays			
1. Describe the attachments and major openings of the diaphragm.	351	361	D13
2. Attachments of respiratory diaphragm.	351	361	J11
3. Major and minor openings of diaphragm.	353	363	J06(RS2), D11(RS3), J19(RS3), J99
Short Answers			
1. Origin of diaphragm.	351	361	D07(RS2)
2. Central tendon of diaphragm.	389	362	D01
3. Openings (major and minor) of diaphragm and structures passing through them.	353	365	J21(RS4), J08(RS2), J09(RS2), D16(RS3), J03, J04, J05, D07
4. Name the structure entering the abdomen under the median, medial and lateral arcuate ligaments.	353	365	J14
5. Structures passing through aortic opening in diaphragm at level of 12th thoracic vertebra.	353	365	D06(RS2), J08, J12
6. Mention the structures passing through the vena caval hiatus of the diaphragm.	353	365	D10
7. Name the structures passing through esophageal opening in diaphragm.	353	365	D11

Contd...

ANATOMY

Contd...

	BDC Vol:2	IBSANT2	
8. Nerve supply of diaphragm.	353	366	J05(RS2), D10(RS2), J98, D03
9. Root value and distribution of phrenic nerve.	353	504	D02
10. Diaphragmatic hernias.	354	367	J12

CHAPTER 57: POSTERIOR ABDOMINAL WALL

Short Essays

1. Abdominal aorta—labeled diagram, branches.	362	456	J06, J10
2. Renal artery and its development.	262	468	D10
3. Inferior vena cava—formation, tributaries and termination.	364	477	J16(RS3), D15
4. Left renal vein.	364	479	D00
5. Iliopsoas.	357	454	J10(RS2)
6. Quadratus lumborum.	357	455	J99, D07
7. Thoracolumbar fascia—layers and attachment.	360	451	F21(RS4), J18(RS3), J03, J12
8. Lumbar plexus—formation and branches.	367	62	D12(RS3), D06, J11
9. Lumbosacral trunk.	367	505	D14

Short Answers

1. Name the branches of abdominal aorta and their level of origin.	362	459	J15(RS3), D14
2. Left renal vein.	364	479	D05(RS2)
3. Tributaries of left renal vein.	365	480	D11
4. Cisterna chyli.	367	483	D14
5. Mention the attachment of thoracolumbar fascia.	360	451	D00
6. Lumbosacral trunk.	367	505	J13(RS3)
7. Celiac plexus.	369	488	J01, D04, J05

Contd...

Contd...

	BDC Vol:2	IBSANT2	
CHAPTER 58: PERINEUM			
Long Essay			
1. Describe ischiorectal (ischioanal) fossa under following headings: (a) Boundaries and recesses; (b) Contents; (c) Applied anatomy.	383	331	D06(RS2), D13(RS3), J00, D08
Short Essays			
1. Perineal body.	381	333	D16(RS3), D98, J02, D04
2. Ischiorectal (ischioanal) fossa—boundaries, contents and applied anatomy.	383	331	J12(RS3), D05(RS2), J09(RS2), J11(RS2), D15(RS3), D16(RS3), D18(RS3), J98, D98, J02, D04, D05, D12, D14, J15
3. Deep perineal pouch—boundaries and contents.	378	328	D19(RS3), D99, J01, J09, D09, D12
4. Perineal membrane—attachments, structures piercing (males and females).	376	329	F21(RS4), D09(RS2), D12(RS3), D17(RS3), D01, D07, D10
5. Urogenital diaphragm.	379	329	J10, J15
6. Describe the attachments and structures piercing the female perineal membrane.	377	329	J14
7. Superficial perineal pouch—boundaries and contents.	377	327	J05(RS2), D10(RS2), J17(RS3), D02, D03, J12, J13

Contd...

Contd...

	BDC Vol:2	IBSANT2	
8. Pudendal canal.	385	333	D05(RS2), J14(RS3), J15(RS3), D02, J07, J09, J10
9. Pudendal nerve.	386	335	J06(RS2), D01, D03
Short Answers			
1. Perineal body (muscles attached).	381	333	D05(RS2), J10(RS2), D15(RS3), J08, D14
2. Ischiorectal (ischioanal) fossa—walls and contents and subdivisions.	383	331	D09, D16
3. Perineal membrane (attachments).	376	329	J12(RS3), D15
4. Why does extravasated urine not enter the thigh under the Colles' fascia?	375	—	D13
5. Urogenital diaphragm—muscles forming and structures piercing.	379	329	J07(RS2), D14(RS3)
6. Perineal muscles.	379	329	D19(RS3)
7. Contents of superficial perineal pouch.	378	327	J09(RS2), D17(RS3), J08
8. Pudendal canal—boundaries and contents.	385	333	F21(RS4), D15
9. Pudendal nerve (course).	386	335	D11(RS3), D12
10. Branches of internal pudendal nerve.	386	335	J07(RS2), D09
11. Pudendal nerve block.	386	337	J05(RS2)
Multiple Choice Questions			
1. Pudendal nerve is the branch of __________. a. Lumbar plexus b. **Sacral plexus** c. Coccygeal plexus d. Lumbosacral trunk	386	335	J21(RS4)

Contd...

Contd...

	BDC Vol:2	IBSANT2	
CHAPTER 59: PRELIMINARY CONSIDERATIONS OF BOUNDARIES AND CONTENTS OF PELVIS			
None.			
CHAPTER 60: URINARY BLADDER AND URETHRA			
Long Essay			
1. Describe urinary bladder under following headings: (a) Position; (b) Capacity; (c) External and internal features; (d) Parts; (e) Surfaces and borders; (f) Peritoneal and visceral relations; (g) Ligaments and supports; (h) The trigone; (i) Blood supply; (j) Nerve supply; (k) Development and congenital anomalies; (l) Applied anatomy.	393	518	J21(RS4), J08(RS2), D09(RS2), D18(RS3), D19(RS3), J98, D15
Short Essays			
1. Urinary bladder—surfaces, labeled diagram, supports, blood supply, nerve supply, lymphatic drainage, development.	393	518	F21(RS4), J07(RS2), J11(RS2), D03, J07, D07, J11
2. Describe the parts, peritoneal relations and interior of the urinary bladder.	395	518	D13
3. Trigone of bladder—boundaries, structure, applied anatomy.	397	523	D15(RS3), J00, J02, J04, D04, D08, J12
4. Nerve supply and development of urinary bladder.	397	524	D10(RS2)
5. Male urethra (parts with their developments).	399	525	D12(RS3), D01, J08
6. Prostatic urethra—length, course, features, structures opening.	401	525	N20(RS3), J98, D98, J01, D07
Short Answers			
1. Supports of urinary bladder.	396	523	D08(RS2)
2. Trigone of urinary bladder.	397	523	D13(RS3), D17(RS3), J15, D16

Contd...

Contd...

	BDC Vol:2	IBSANT2	
3. Nerve supply of urinary bladder.	397	524	J15(RS3), N20(RS3), D11
4. Male urethra—parts.	399	525	D18(RS3)
5. Which is the most dilatable part of the male urethra? Mentions structures opening in it.	401	525	J21(RS4)
6. Prostatic urethra.	401	525	D15(RS3), J17(RS3), J18(RS3), D14

CHAPTER 61: FEMALE REPRODUCTIVE ORGANS

Long Essays

1. Describe uterus under following headings: (a) Position (normal axis) and parts; (b) Gross anatomy; (c) Peritoneal reflections; (d) Relations; (e) Supports; (f) Blood supply; (g) Development; (h) Applied anatomy.	415	538	J05(RS2), J06(RS2), J11(RS2), J19(RS3), N20(RS3), J99, D99, J03, D05, J13, D14

Short Essays

1. Ovarian fossa.	409	535	J00
2. Ovary—position, parts, surfaces, relations, ligaments, blood supply.	409	534	J01, D06, J07, J12, D16
3. Ovary—relations and histology.	410	535	D12(RS3)
4. Fallopian/uterine tube (parts, blood supply, applied aspects and development).	413	536	J21(RS4), D13(RS3), D18(RS3), J99, D01, D03, D05, J06, D10
5. Name the parts of the uterus and explain the supports of the uterus.	420	539	J14
6. Ligaments of uterus.	417	541	J05
7. Broad ligament of uterus—attachments and contents.	417	542	J04, D09
8. Uterus—blood supply and lymphatic drainage.	417	545	D08

Contd...

Contd...

	BDC Vol:2	IBSANT2	
9. Supports of uterus and their applied importance.	420	543	J08(RS2), D17(RS3), J18(RS3), D00, J02, D04, D07, D10, D15
Short Answers			
1. Ovarian fossa (relations).	409	535	J10, J14, J15
2. Mesovarium.	410	535	J11
3. Fallopian (uterine) tube—parts and blood supply.	413	536	J06(RS2), D99, D09, D16
4. Enumerate the parts of uterus and fallopian tube.	413, 415	539, 536	D12(RS3)
5. Tubectomy.	415	538	D11(RS3), J08
6. Positions and parts of uterus.	416	538	D06(RS2)
7. Normal position of uterus.	416	540	J11
8. Uterine axis.	416	540	J14(RS3)
9. Name the ligaments attached to the cervix of the uterus.	417	541	D16
10. Broad ligament of uterus—contents.	418	542	J05(RS2), D16(RS3), D12
11. Course and branches of uterine artery.	418	502	J14(RS3)
12. Four supports of uterus.	420	543	J15
13. Uterosacral ligament.	421	543	J13(RS3)
14. Vagina.	423	545	J13(RS3)
Multiple Choice Questions			
1. The angle of anteflexion of uterus is________. a. 45° b. 60° c. 90° d. **125°**	415	540	J21(RS4)

Contd...

ANATOMY

Contd...

	BDC Vol:2	IBSANT2	
CHAPTER 62: MALE REPRODUCTIVE ORGANS			
Long Essay			
1. Describe prostate gland under following headings: (a) Coverings (capsule); (b) Parts (lobes); (c) Relations; (d) Blood supply; (e) Age changes; (f) Applied anatomy (surgical importance).	429	530	J09(RS2), D11(RS3)
Short Essays			
1. Prostate—location (position), capsule (coverings), lobes (parts), blood supply, age changes and applied anatomy.	429	530	D05(RS2), D06(RS2), D09(RS2), J13(RS3), D19(RS3), D00, J06, D06, J14, D16
2. Lobes of prostate gland.	431	530	D14(RS3), D15(RS3)
Short Answers			
1. Vas deferens.	424	529	J09(RS2)
2. Vasectomy.	428	324	D00
CHAPTER 63: RECTUM AND ANAL CANAL			
Long Essays			
1. Describe rectum and anal canal under the following headings: (a) Gross anatomy; (b) Supports; (c) Blood supply.	436, 441	508, 514	D10
2. Describe interior of rectum and anal canal. Add a note on it's (a) Development; and (b) Applied anatomy.	437, 441	509, 515	D08(RS2)
3. Describe anal canal under following headings: (a) Extent; (b) Development/embryological origin; (c) Gross anatomy; (d) Internal features; (e) Sphincters; (f) Blood supply; (g) Lymphatic drainage; (h) Nerve supply; (i) Applied anatomy.	441	514	J16(RS3), J17(RS3), J18(RS3), D02, J11

Contd...

Contd...

	BDC Vol:2	IBSANT2	
Short Essays			
1. Rectum—extent, relations	436	508	J07
2. Blood supply and development of rectum and anal canal.	438, 444	512, 517	J01
3. Anal canal—location, interior, blood supply, lymphatic drainage and development.	441	514	J07(RS2), D09(RS2), D98, J99, J06, D06, D09, D11
4. Describe the interior of the anal canal and add a note on its applied anatomy.	441	515	J19(RS3), J13, D13
Short Answers			
1. Valves present in the rectum/What are Houston's valves and what is its function?	437	509	D12, D16
2. Rectum—peritoneal relations and their clinical importance.	437	510	F21(RS4)
3. Pectinate line/Hilton's line—importance.	442	515	D12(RS3), J13(RS3)
4. Anal sphincters.	442	515	D13(RS3)
5. Sphincter ani externus muscle.	442	515	D07
6. Name the causes and types of hemorrhoids in the anal canal.	445	517	D12, J14

CHAPTER 64: WALLS OF PELVIS

Short Essays			
1. Internal iliac artery—origin, course, branches and area of distribution.	452	500	J21(RS4), J15(RS3), D00
2. Describe the branches of the anterior trunk of the internal iliac artery.	452	500	D13
3. Nervi erigentis.	457	—	J03
4. Levator ani muscle.	449	496	J12(RS3), J03

Contd...

ANATOMY

Contd...

	BDC Vol:2	IBSANT2	
5. Pelvic diaphragm—components, attachment of muscles, openings, functions.	451	496	J13(RS3), J14(RS3), D19(RS3), N20(RS3), J04, D06
6. Sacrotuberous ligament.	458	227	D11
Short Answers			
1. Branches of external iliac artery.	—	473	J06
2. Branches of internal iliac artery.	452	500	J05(RS2), D13(RS3), D08
3. Name the branches of the anterior division of the internal iliac artery.	452	500	D12
4. Name the branches of posterior trunk of internal iliac artery.	452	500	D14
5. Nervi erigentis.	457	—	J06
6. What are the different components of the levator ani muscle?	450	496	D16
7. What are the different components of the pelvic diaphragm?	451	496	D12
8. Name the muscles forming the pelvic diaphragm.	451	496	D11
9. Sacrotuberous ligament—attachments and morphology.	458	227	D05(RS2)

	BDC Vol:3	IBSANT3	
SECTION 6: HEAD AND NECK			
CHAPTER 65: OSTEOLOGY OF HEAD AND NECK			
Short Essays			
1. Superior orbital fissure.	22, 24	20, 39	N20(RS3), J05
2. Hyoid bone.	46	50	J07(RS2), J00, J03
Short Answers			
1. Name paired bones of cranium.	2	—	J10

Contd...

Contd...

	BDC Vol:3	IBSANT3	
2. Anterior fontanelle and its clinical importance.	4	45	J08
3. Bregma—labeled diagram.	4	18	J06
4. Nasion.	6	20	D17(RS3)
5. Asterion—bones meeting and venous sinus related deep to it.	10	26	D02
6. Pterion—bone meeting and its clinical importance.	11	25	D14(RS3), J00, J01, D04, J07
7. Attachments of mastoid process.	10	28	D03
8. Hard palate—bones forming.	11	131	J12(RS3), J18(RS3), J05
9. Superior orbital fissure—boundaries and structures passing through (contents).	22, 24	20, 39	J06(RS2), D06, J09
10. Foramen spinosum.	24	41	D16
11. Mention two features of the fetal skull.	28	—	D10
12. Name foramina in middle cranial fossa.	18	40	D06(RS2)
13. Foramen ovale—structures passing through.	18	40	D11(RS3), J16(RS3), J05, J07, J08, J12
14. Foramen magnum—structures passing through.	19	41	J11(RS2), J18(RS3), D99, J04
15. Jugular foramen—structure passing through.	19	41	J02, D09

CHAPTER 66: SCALP, TEMPLE AND FACE

Long Essays

1. Define and name layers of the scalp. Give its blood supply, nerve supply and applied anatomy.	54	65	J10(RS2), D00
2. Describe blood supply and venous drainage of face and add a note on applied anatomy.	75	83	D05(RS2)

Contd...

Contd...

	BDC Vol:3	IBSANT3	
Short Essays			
1. Scalp—layers, blood supply and nerve supply/Applied anatomy.	54	65	D07(RS2), D14(RS3), J15(RS3), D15(RS3), D16(RS3), D08
2. Emissary veins.	57	354	J03
3. Orbicularis oculi—parts, attachments, nerve supply and actions.	62	80	D06(RS2), J13(RS3)
4. Buccinator muscle.	62	80	J15(RS3), J03, D14
5. Cutaneous innervation of face.	65	85	J08(RS2)
6. Facial artery in face	66	326	N20(RS3)
7. Lacrimal apparatus.	71	75	J11(RS2), D15(RS3), D16
Short Answers			
1. Name the layers of scalp and mention the dangerous layer of scalp.	54	65	D06, D11, D14
2. Retromandibular vein (formation).	57	347	J16(RS3), J99
3. Sensory nerve supply of scalp.	57	68	J11
4. Nerves supplying (sensory and motor innervations) anterior quadrant of scalp.	57	68	J14
5. What is black eye? Explain the anatomical basis of 'black eye'.	58	67	J21(RS4), J12(RS3), J00, J09
6. Buccinator muscle.	62	80	D07(RS2)
7. Platysma.	62	185	J09
8. Features of Bell's palsy.	64	86	J05(RS2)
9. Sensory nerve supply of face.	65	85	J13(RS3), D99
10. Facial vein.	67	83	D17(RS3)

Contd...

Contd...

	BDC Vol:3	IBSANT3	
11. Dangerous area of the face.	68	83	D16(RS3), D19(RS3), J13
12. Constituents of lacrimal apparatus and their function.	71	75	D06, J13
13. Nasolacrimal duct.	73	77	D13(RS3), J16(RS3), J11

CHAPTER 67: SIDE OF NECK

Long Essay			
1. Describe the boundaries, parts and contents of posterior triangle of neck.	83	197	D12(RS3), J19(RS3), J07
Short Essays			
1. General investing layer of deep cervical fascia.	76	177	J18(RS3), J03
2. Carotid sheath.	80	180	D08(RS2), J11(RS2), D17(RS3), D99, J00, D03
3. External jugular vein—formation, relations, tributaries and applied anatomy.	84	344	J10
Short Answers			
1. Virchow's node.	—	—	D06
2. Fascia—Colles'.	76	176	J11
3. Suprasternal space (of Burn)—contents.	77	—	J19(RS3), J12
4. Pretracheal fascia.	79	178	D10(RS2)
5. Suspensory ligament of Berry.	79	178	J07
6. Prevertebral fascia—attachments and extensions.	79	180	F21(RS4)
7. Contents of carotid sheath.	80	180	J05(RS2), J07(RS2), J11

Contd...

Contd...

	BDC Vol:3	IBSANT3	
8. Sternocleidomastoid muscle—origin, insertion, nerve supply and actions.	81	185	N20(RS3), D99, J15
9. Torticollis (wry neck).	82	188	J01, D04
10. External jugular vein—formation, termination and tributaries.	84	344	D13(RS3), D14(RS3), J15(RS3), J00, J12, D13, D16

CHAPTER 68: ANTERIOR TRIANGLE OF NECK

Short Essays

1. Diagastric triangle—boundaries and contents.	94	202	J18(RS3), D08
2. Carotid triangle.	96	204	J09
3. Ansa cervicalis—formation, labeled diagram, distribution.	98	418	J15(RS3), J16(RS3), D98, D05
4. Carotid sinus.	99	311	D09
5. Describe the origin, course, branches and termination of the external carotid artery.	99	321	J13
6. Lingual artery.	100	325	D09(RS2)
7. Facial artery—origin, termination, course, relation and branches.	101	326	J09(RS2), J06, D07, J09

Short Answers

1. Digastric triangle (contents).	94	202	J10(RS2), D98, D14
2. Draw a neat labeled diagram of boundaries and subdivisions of anterior triangle of neck.	94	201	J15(RS3)
3. Boundaries and contents of carotid triangle.	96	204	J14(RS3), J14
4. Boundaries of muscular triangles of neck.	98	201	D06
5. Ansa cervicalis (root value, branches and distribution).	98	418	J11(RS2), J15

Contd...

Contd...

	BDC Vol:3	IBSANT3	
6. (Six) branches of external carotid artery.	100	322	F21(RS4), J06(RS2), J17(RS3), J18(RS3), J98, D08, D11, J15
7. Facial artery (branches).	101	326	J13(RS3), J05

CHAPTER 69: PAROTID REGION

Long Essay

1. Describe parotid salivary gland under following headings: (a) Position; (b) Surfaces, borders, relations and duct; (c) Coverings; (d) Parts; (e) Contents (structures passing through within it); (f) Blood and nerve supply; (g) Applied anatomy.	103	88	D19(RS3), D03, D07, J11, D11, J14

Short Essays

1. Parotid gland (nerve supply).	107	88	J09
2. Parotid duct—origin, termination, relations and structures pierced by it.	108	94	J06(RS2), J01, D05, J07

Short Answers

1. Structures present within substance of parotid gland.	107	92	J09(RS2), J02, D08
2. Trace pathway for secretomotor (parasympathetic) fibers to parotid gland.	107	95	J98, J10, D12
3. Parotid duct (Stenson's duct).	108	94	D05(RS2), D08(RS2), D98, D16
4. Structure pierced by parotid duct before its termination.	108	95	D99

Contd...

Contd...

	BDC Vol:3	IBSANT3	
CHAPTER 70: TEMPORAL AND INFRATEMPORAL FOSSA			
Long Essays			
1. Name muscles of mastication. Describe them under following headings: (a) Origin; (b) Insertion; (c) Nerve supply; (d) Actions. Add a note on its development.	113	99	J08(RS2), J11(RS2), D13(RS3), D18(RS3), D14
2. Describe temporomandibular joint under following headings: (a) Formation; (b) Ligaments; (c) Relations; (d) Movements and muscles causing it; (e) Applied anatomy.	120	111	J19(RS3), D01, D10
Short Essays			
1. Temporalis—attachments, nerve supply, action.	114	99	J12(RS3), J04
2. Lateral pterygoid muscle and its relations.	114	99	D05(RS2), J17(RS3), N20(RS3), D00
3. Maxillary artery.	117	107	J02, D04
4. Articular disc of temporomandibular joint.	121	113	J00
5. Movements of temporomandibular joint and muscles causing them.	122	114	D10(RS2), D15(RS3)
6. Lingual nerve—origin, course and distribution.	125	126	D12
7. Otic ganglion and its connections.	126	422	J05(RS2), D17(RS3), J99, J03, J11
Short Answers			
1. Muscles of mastication and their nerve supply.	114	99	J15
2. Lateral pterygoid muscle—nerve supply and actions.	114	99	J10
3. Branches of maxillary artery—1st part/3rd part.	118	107	J05, D07, J14
4. Ligaments of temporomandibular joint.	120	113	D06

Contd...

Contd...

	BDC Vol:3	IBSANT3	
5. Movements of protraction and retraction of mandible.	122	114	J07(RS2)
6. Branches of mandibular nerve.	124	388	D01
7. Enumerate the muscles supplied by mandibular nerve.	125	388	J12
8. Auriculotemporal nerves.	125	389	D15(RS3)
Multiple Choice Questions			
1. All the following are muscles elevates jaw, *except*: a. Temporalis b. **Lateral pterygoid** c. Medial pterygoid d. Masseter	114	114	J21(RS4)

CHAPTER 71: SUBMANDIBULAR REGION

Short Essays			
1. Hyoglossus muscle.	130	143	J09(RS2), J98, J01, D03, D06, J15, D15
2. Submandibular salivary gland—location, parts, relations and nerve supply.	132	120	J13, D15
3. Submandibular ganglion.	135	422	D12(RS3)
Short Answers			
1. Digastric muscle—origin, insertion and nerve supply.	130	125	D10(RS2), J00
2. Submandibular duct.	134	122	D15(RS3), D12
3. Mention the secretomotor supply of submandibular salivary gland.	134	123	D10, J15
4. Submandibular ganglion.	135	422	D09
5. Secretomotor fibers of submandibular ganglion.	135	422	D14(RS3)
Multiple Choice Questions			
1. Presynaptic parasympathetic secretomotor fibers to submandibular gland relays in: a. Trigeminal ganglion b. **Submandibular ganglion** c. Sphenopalatine ganglion d. Otic ganglion	135	123	J21(RS4)

Contd...

Contd...

	BDC Vol:3	IBSANT3	
CHAPTER 72: STRUCTURES IN THE NECK			
Long Essays			
1. Describe thyroid gland under following headings: (a) Position; (b) Parts; (c) Capsule and ligaments; (d) Gross features; (e) Relations; (f) Blood supply and venous drainage; (g) Histology (microscopic anatomy); (h) Development; (i) Applied anatomy. Explain the anatomical basis of movement of the thyroid gland in the anterior midline with deglutition.	138	303	J21(RS4), D06(RS2), D10(RS2), D11(RS3), J13(RS3), D16(RS3), J17(RS3), N20(RS3), J99, D02, J03
Short Essays			
1. Describe the position, parts, relations and coverings of the thyroid gland.	138	303	D18(RS3), D13
2. Thyroid gland—blood supply.	140	306	D11
3. Parathyroid glands.	144	308	J01, J05
4. Internal jugular vein (tributaries).	153	341	D01
5. Submandibular group of lymph nodes.	159	356	D02
6. Styloid apparatus.	161	—	J99, J04, D08
Short Answers			
1. Labeled diagram of thyroid gland.	138	304	J05
2. Thyroid gland—blood supply and venous drainage.	140	306	D15(RS3), D08
3. Blood supply to isthmus of thyroid.	141	307	J07(RS2)
4. Internal jugular vein—tributaries.	153	343	J05(RS2), J10(RS2), D09, J15
5. Name the tributaries of the left brachiocephalic vein.	154	489 (IBSANT1)	D10
6. Features of Horner's syndrome.	158	422	J12(RS3), D18(RS3), D01
7. Styloid apparatus.	161	—	J14(RS3), J19(RS3)

Contd...

ANATOMY

Contd...

	BDC Vol:3	IBSANT3	
8. Styloid process of temporal bone.	161	27	D05(RS2), D15(RS3)

CHAPTER 73: PREVERTEBRAL AND PARAVERTEBRAL REGION

Short Essays

1. Trachea.	166	245	D02
2. Atlantoaxial joint.	173	59	D99
3. Describe the movements that occur at the atlanto-occipital and median atlantoaxial joints and the muscles causing them. Explain the mechanism by which movements occur at the median atlantoaxial joint.	173	61	F21(RS4)

Short Answers

1. Type and movements at atalanto-occipital joint.	173	60	J02
2. Cervical pleura.	—	—	D03

CHAPTER 74: BACK OF NECK

Short Essays

1. Suboccipital space (triangle)—boundaries and contents.	183	205	J06(RS2), D11(RS3)
2. Suboccipital nerve.	185	416	J09

Short Answers

1. Suboccipital triangle.	183	205	J08(RS2), D09(RS2)
2. Suboccipital nerve.	185	416	J01, D04

CHAPTER 75: CONTENTS OF VERTEBRAL CANAL

Short Essays

1. Filum terminale.	188	172	J12

Contd...

Contd...

	BDC Vol:3	IBSANT3	
2. A lumbar puncture was done on a 6-year-old boy who was suspected to have tubercular meningitis. a. Name the meningeal layers and spaces that cover the brain and spinal cord. b. In which space is the cerebrospinal fluid present? c. Explain the anatomical basis of the selection of the site of lumbar puncture. d. Name the structures traversed by the needle from superficial to deep before it reaches the space while performing the lumbar puncture.	188	174	J21(RS4)
3. Cauda equina.	190	173	D02
Short Answers			
1. Modifications of pia mater.	188	172	D16
2. Ligamentum denticulatum.	188	172	D10(RS2), J17(RS3)
3. Filum terminale.	188	172	J11(RS2), D11(RS3), J18(RS3), J06, D12
4. Lumbar puncture at L3/L4 interspinous level—anatomical basis.	188	174	F21(RS4)
5. Cauda equina.	190	173	D08, D16

CHAPTER 76: CRANIAL CAVITY

Long Essay			
1. Classify dural venous sinuses. Describe cavernous sinus under following headings: (a) Relations; (b) Tributaries; (c) Communications; (d) Applied anatomy.	196	348, 351	J05(RS2), J18(RS3), J98, J02, D06, J10, D13, D16
Short Essays			
1. Falx cerebri.	194	160	D08(RS2), D14

Contd...

Contd...

	BDC Vol:3	IBSANT3	
2. Cavernous sinus—situation, tributaries and structures within. How can infection spread into the cavernous sinus?	196	351	J21(RS4), J07(RS2), D08(RS2), J08
3. Pituitary gland—position, parts and secretions.	201	298	D12
Short Answers			
1. Name the cranial dural folds.	194	159	J13
2. Falx cerebri.	194	160	D06(RS2), J11
3. Venous sinuses present in falx cerebri.	195	160	J06
4. Tentorium cerebelli.	195	162	N20(RS3)
5. Name the dural venous sinuses related to tentorium cerebella.	195	162	D14
6. Name paired dural venous sinuses.	196	348	D11
7. Name the structures present in the lateral wall of the cavernous sinus.	197	352	J13
8. Cavernous sinus—tributaries of cavernous sinus.	197	352	D05(RS2), J04
9. Superior sagittal sinus.	200	348	D12(RS3)
10. Straight sinus—formation, termination and applied anatomy.	200	349	D11(RS3), J07, D09
11. Sigmoid sinus.	201	351	D09(RS2), D12
12. Blood supply of hypophysis.	202	302	D07(RS2)
13. What is hypothalamohypophysial portal system?	203	302	J14
Multiple Choice Questions			
1. The dural venous sinus present in the free border of falx cerebri is: a. **Inferior sagittal sinus** b. Superior sagittal sinus c. Transverse sinus d. Straight sinus	194	162	J21(RS4)

Contd...

Contd...

	BDC Vol:3	IBSANT3	
CHAPTER 77: CONTENTS OF THE ORBIT			
Long Essay			
1. Describe extraocular muscles under following headings: (a) Origin; (b) Insertion; (c) Relations; (d) Actions; (e) Nerve supply; (f) Applied anatomy. Discuss the movements of eyeball.	211	256	J15(RS3), D17(RS3), J04, J05, J09, J15
Short Essays			
1. Explain the attachments, action and nerve supply of the recti muscles of the eyeball.	212	256	J14
2. Oblique muscles of eyeball, their origin, insertion, action and nerve supply.	212	256	D16(RS3)
3. Ciliary ganglion—type, location, connections (roots, branches).	218	422	D10(RS2), J13(RS3), D00, D01, J04, D07, D11, D16
Short Answers			
1. Name extraocular muscles and give their nerve supply.	211	256	J02, D13, D15
2. Lateral rectus muscle of eye.	212	256	J11
3. Superior oblique muscle of the eye (nerve supply and action).	212	256	J10(RS2), J99, J10, D12
4. Levator palpebrae superioris (nerve supply).	212	256	D15(RS3)
5. Nerve supply and actions of inferior rectus muscle of eyeball.	213	256	D14
6. Ciliary ganglion (secretomotor fibers).	218	422	J16(RS3)
CHAPTER 78: MOUTH AND PHARYNX			
Long Essays			
1. Describe muscles, nerve supply, development and congenital anomalies of soft palate.	229	133	D09

Contd...

Contd...

	BDC Vol:3	IBSANT3	
2. Name the muscles of the soft palate. Give: (a) Origin; (b) Insertion; (c) Nerve supply of levator veli palatine muscle. Describe the movements of soft palate. Add a note on development of soft palate.	229	133	J09(RS2)
3. Name the different types of tonsils. Describe Palatine Tonsil under following headings: (a) Position; (b) Blood supply; (c) Relations; (d) Microscopic anatomy; (e) Development; (f) Applied anatomy.	242	152	J12(RS3)
4. Name the muscles of pharynx. Give (a) Origin; (b) Insertion; (c) Nerve supply; (d) Actions; (e) Relations of superior constrictor muscle of pharynx. Add a note on its surgical anatomy.	245	231	D07(RS2)
Short Essays			
1. Soft palate.	229	131	J99
2. Describe the attachment, actions and nerve supply of the muscles of soft palate. Explain the role of the soft palate in deglutition.	229, 232	133	F21(RS4), D11(RS3), J13
3. Mention the subdivisions of the pharynx and explain the nasopharynx.	234	224	J13
4. Nasopharynx.	234	226	D02
5. Palatine tonsil—relations, blood supply and applied anatomy.	229	153	J10, D12
6. Muscles of pharynx.	245	231	J08(RS2)
7. Constrictors of pharynx.	245	231	J12
8. Inferior constrictor of pharynx.	245	232	D08
9. Auditory tube—length, extent, relations and functions.	244	286	J98, J02, D04, D07
Short Answers			
1. Location and content of the tubal tonsil.	—	228	D13
2. Openings in nasopharynx.	—	228	J05

Contd...

Contd...

	BDC Vol:3	IBSANT3	
3. Name muscles of soft palate with nerve supply.	229	133	J10, D15
4. Structures forming Waldeyer's ring.	241	153	J01, D04, D07
5. Tonsillar bed.	229	154	D19(RS3)
6. Blood supply and lymphatic drainage of tonsil.	230	155	D09(RS2), J99, D14
7. Killian's dehiscence.	240	233	J09
8. Nerve supply of pharynx.	240	234	J04
9. Give the dimensions and functions of auditory tube.	245	288	J12
10. Location of openings of auditory tube.	245	288	D05

CHAPTER 79: NOSE AND PARANASAL SINUSES

Short Essays

1. Nasal septum—formation, blood supply and nerve supply.	247	212	D07(RS2), J17(RS3), D19(RS3), N20(RS3), J08, J10, J12, D14
2. Lateral wall of nasal cavity—features, blood supply and innervations.	248	215	J14(RS3), J05, D10, D13, J14
3. Middle meatus of nose.	250	218	D05(RS2)
4. Maxillary air sinus.	252	221	J05(RS2), J06(RS2), D11
5. Pterygopalatine ganglion.	256	422	J10(RS2)

Short Answers

1. Components of nasal septum.	247	212	J14
2. Blood supply of nasal septum.	247	214	J10(RS2)
3. What is Little's area of the nose? Explain its clinical importance.	247	214	J21(RS4), D16
4. Name the bones that contribute to the lateral wall of the nasal cavity. Explain the functional importance of the turbinates.	250	215	F21(RS4)

Contd...

Contd...

	BDC Vol:3	IBSANT3	
5. Middle meatus of nose (osteomeatal complex).	250	218	D18(RS3), D98, D03
6. Structures opening in middle meatus of nose.	251	218	D06(RS2), J08, D09, D16
7. Name the paranasal air sinuses opening into middle meatus of nose.	251	218	D15
8. Frontal sinus.	252	221	D17(RS3)
9. Maxillary sinus.	252	221	D14(RS3)
10. Pterygopalatine fossa—contents.	280	384	D02
11. Pterygopalatine ganglion.	256	422	J09

CHAPTER 80: LARYNX

Long Essays

1. Describe the cartilages and muscles of larynx.	259	236	D15(RS3)
2. Describe the larynx under the following headings: (a) Cavity; (b) Actions of intrinsic muscles; (c) Nerve supply. Explain the anatomical basis of injuries to the nerves supplying the larynx during thyroid surgeries.	262	241	F21(RS4)
3. Describe the intrinsic muscles of larynx with applied aspects.	264	244	D14(RS3)
4. Name intrinsic muscles of larynx. Give (a) Origin; (b) Insertion; (c) Nerve supply; (d) Actions of cricothyroid muscle. Add a note on movements of vocal cords.	264	244	D08(RS2)

Short Essays

1. Thyroid cartilage.	259	236	J15(RS3)
2. Interior (cavity) of larynx.	262	241	D18(RS3), D15
3. Vocal cords (folds).	262	241	J98, J01, D07
4. Muscles of larynx.	264	244	J11
5. Cricothyroid muscle.	265	244	D98

Contd...

Contd...

	BDC Vol:3	IBSANT3	
Short Answers			
1. Epiglottis.	260	238	D05(RS2)
2. Inlet of larynx.	263	241	D12(RS3)
3. Rima glottidis (parts and muscles which open it).	263	242	J02
4. Piriform/pyriform fossa—boundaries and applied importance.	264	230	D13
5. Enumerate only intrinsic muscles of larynx.	264	244	J09
6. Cricothyroid muscle—nerve supply and action.	264	244	D10
7. Posterior cricoarytenoids—nerve supply and actions.	264	244	D01, D12
8. Name the abductors of vocal cord.	264	245	D16(RS3)
9. Larynx—nerve supply (sensory and motor).	267	243	J06(RS2), D10(RS2), D02, D03, J05, J14
Multiple Choice Questions			
1. All the following cartilages are unpaired, *except*: a. Thyroid b. Cricoid c. **Corniculate** d. Epiglottis	259	236	J21(RS4)

CHAPTER 81: TONGUE

Long Essays			
1. Describe the tongue under following headings: (a) Parts; (b) Gross anatomy; (c) Dorsum of tongue; (d) Muscle; (e) Nerve supply; (f) Blood Supply; (g) Lymphatic drainage; (h) Development; (i) Applied anatomy.	271	138	D98, J00, D08, J12
2. Name muscles of tongue. Give (a) Origin; (b) Insertion; (c) Nerve supply; (d) Actions. Add a note on its development.	272	141	D09(RS2)

Contd...

Contd...

	BDC Vol:3	IBSANT3	
Short Essays			
1. Name the muscles of the tongue and explain their actions and nerve supply.	272	141	D12
2. Tongue—lymphatic drainage.	273	150	D08(RS2), D12(RS3)
3. Tongue—lymphatic drainage and development.	273	150	J11(RS2)
4. Tongue—development and nerve supply.	273	145	D16(RS3), D19(RS3)
5. Tongue—sensory and motor nerve supply.	273	145	D06(RS2), D01, J15
Short Answers			
1. Tongue—innervation/nerve supply (sensory).	273	145	J08(RS2), J09(RS2), D15(RS3), D13
2. Tongue—lymphatic drainage	273	150	N20(RS3)
CHAPTER 82: EAR			
Long Essay			
1. Describe the medial and lateral walls of middle ear and add a note on its applied aspects.	284	279	D15
Short Essays			
1. Tympanic membrane.	281	279	D09(RS2), D98, D00, J12, D12
2. Tympanic cavity.	283	276	D03
3. Walls of middle ear.	284	279	D13(RS3)
4. Posterior wall of middle ear.	284	281	D07(RS2)
5. Lateral wall of middle ear.	284	279	J12(RS3)
6. Medial wall of middle ear.	284	282	J07, J10
Short Answers			
1. Name the components and medial relations of the tympanic membrane.	281	279	J13

Contd...

Contd...

	BDC Vol:3	IBSANT3	
2. A 50-year-old man presented with severe ear pain because of the rupture of his tympanic membrane following an accidental injury. Explain the nerve supply of the tympanic membrane.	282	280	J21(RS4)
3. Draw only medial wall of middle ear cavity.	285	283	J09
4. Contents of middle ear.	287	283	J00, D01

CHAPTER 83: EYEBALL

Short Essays

1. Cornea.	296	264	D05(RS2)

Short Answer

1. Name the muscles of the eyeball.	298	267	D10

CHAPTER 84: MISCELLANEOUS

None

	BDC Vol:4	IBSANT3	
SECTION 7: BRAIN			

CHAPTER 85: INTRODUCTION

None.

CHAPTER 86: MENINGES OF BRAIN AND CEREBROSPINAL FLUID

Short Essay

1. Subarachnoid cisterns.	26	166	J15(RS3)

Short Answer

1. Mention function of arachnoid granulations.	25	167	D05

Contd...

ANATOMY

Contd...

	BDC Vol:4	IBSANT3	
CHAPTER 87: SPINAL CORD			
Short Essay			
1. Draw a neat, labeled diagram of the cross-section of the spinal cord at the mid-thoracic level showing ascending and descending tracts. Explain the functional importance of the dorsal columns.	35, 39	481, 490	F21(RS4), J07
Short Answers			
1. Cross section of spinal cord to show ascending and descending tracts (only labeled diagram).	35, 39	481	D05(RS2)
2. Sensation carried by posterior column of spinal cord.	39	490	D06
CHAPTER 88: CRANIAL NERVES			
Long Essays			
1. Describe occulomotor nerve under following headings: (a) Origin; (b) Course; (c) Relations; (d) Distribution; (e) Applied anatomy.	58	373	D02, D04
2. Describe facial nerve under following headings: (a) Origin; (b) Course; (c) Relations; (d) Distribution.	66	393	J08
Short Essays			
1. Describe the extracranial course, distribution of the facial nerve.	67	395	D12
2. Facial nerve in face.	67	395	J05
3. Left recurrent laryngeal nerve.	78	410	D99
Short Answers			
1. Enumerate the cranial nerves taking origin from medulla oblongata.	49	465	D14
2. Accommodation reflex.	56	—	D13(RS3)
3. Muscles supplied by third cranial (oculomotor) nerve.	59	373	D99

Contd...

Contd...

	BDC Vol:4	IBSANT3	
4. Muscles affected in oculomotor palsy.	59	373	D06(RS2)
5. Name the branches of the trigeminal nerve in the face.	63	379	J13
6. Branches of facial nerve on face.	67	397	D07
7. Nerve to stapedius.	68	396	J07(RS2)
8. Chorda tympani nerve (structures supplied).	68	398	J15(RS3), D05, J09
9. Branches of hypoglossal nerve.	82	415	D09
Multiple Choice Questions			
1. Deviation of tongue to affected side due to unilateral hypoglossal nerve injury is because of: a. Affected genioglossus muscle on the other side b. Unaffected palatoglossus muscle on the other side c. **Unaffected genioglossus muscle on the other side** d. Affected palatoglossus muscle on the same side	82	416	J21(RS4)
CHAPTER 89: BRAINSTEM			
Long Essays			
1. Draw a diagram of transverse section of medulla oblongata at sensory decussation and label parts.	89	468	J98
Short Essays			
1. Transverse section of medulla at various levels.	89	466	D16
2. Describe (draw a neat labeled diagram) the cross-section of medulla oblongata at the level of sensory decussation.	89	467	J21(RS4), D15(RS3), J16(RS3), D03, J07
3. Draw and label the transverse section of medulla oblongata at the pyramidal decussation.	89	467	J12(RS3), D13(RS3), J00, J10, D15
4. Pontine nuclei—location, connections.	91	471	J06

Contd...

Contd...

	BDC Vol:4	IBSANT3	
5. Section of pons at midlevel.	93	471	J04
6. Medial lemniscus.	94	476	D05(RS2)
7. Midbrain.	94	474	J09(RS2), J10(RS2)
8. Transverse section of midbrain at level of inferior colliculus (draw and label).	96	475	D07(RS2), D12(RS3), D14(RS3), D07
9. Labeled diagram showing transverse section of midbrain at level of superior colliculus. Add a note on connections of red nucleus.	97	476	J05(RS2), J06(RS2), J08(RS2), J13(RS3), D00, J13
10. Superior colliculus.	96	476	D17(RS3)
11. Red nucleus—location, connections.	96	476	D11(RS3), J16(RS3), J99, J08, J12
Short Answers			
1. Nucleus ambiguus.	88	502	J14(RS3)
2. Crus cerebri.	96	474	D16(RS3)
3. Draw transverse section of midbrain at inferior colliculus.	96	475	D09
4. Red nucleus.	96	476	J17(RS3)

CHAPTER 90: CEREBELLUM

Short Essays

1. Cerebellum—parts of vermis (divisions) and its functions.	101	511	J14(RS3), D09
2. Nuclei of cerebellum.	103	516	J19(RS3)
3. Dentate nucleus—situation, shape, connections and functions.	103	516	J02, D04, D07
4. Cerebellar peduncles.	104	518	J07(RS2)
5. Superior cerebellar peduncle.	104	519	J15

Contd...

ANATOMY

Contd...

	BDC Vol:4	IBSANT3	
6. Inferior cerebellar peduncle—parts connected, fibers passing through.	104	518	D06(RS2), J09(RS2), J13(RS3), D14(RS3), D99, J00, D02, J04, D08
7. Functions and applied anatomy of cerebellum.	106	517	J10, D11
Short Answers			
1. Archicerebellum.	101	512	D08(RS2)
2. Enumerate nuclei of cerebellum.	103	516	J10(RS2)
3. Mention any two afferent and efferent fibers present in the middle cerebral peduncle.	104	518	J14
4. Name the tracts in inferior cerebellar peduncle.	104	520	J11
Multiple Choice Questions			
1. Which one of the following is not an intracerebellar nucleus? a. **Vestibular** b. Dentate c. Fastigii d. Globosus	103	516	J21(RS4)

CHAPTER 91: FOURTH VENTRICLE

Short Essays			
1. Fourth ventricle—boundaries.	109	561	D19(RS3), D13
2. Floor of 4th ventricle (labeled diagram).	109	562	J12(RS3), J06(RS2), D16(RS3), J99, J11, D11, D12
3. Rhomboid fossa (4th ventricle).	109	562	D09(RS2), J18(RS3), D16
Short Answers			
1. Rhomboid fossa—boundaries.	109	561	J09

Contd...

Contd...

	BDC Vol:4	IBSANT3	
2. Draw a neat labeled diagram of the floor of the fourth (IV) ventricle.	109	562	J21(RS4)
3. Roof of 4th ventricle.	111	563	D08(RS2)
4. Formation and function of the tela choroidia.	112	560	D13
5. What is cerebral aqueduct? And what is its clinical importance?	112	—	D13

CHAPTER 92: CEREBRUM

Long Essays

1. Describe the superolateral surface of cerebral hemisphere under the following headings: (a) Lobes; (b) Sulci; (c) Gyri; (d) Functional areas; (e) Blood supply.	129	529	J13(RS3), J14(RS3), J01
2. Describe thalamus and its connections.	114	537	D09
3. Describe the extent, gross features and relations of the hypothalamus. Explain the functional importance of the hypothalamic-hypophyseal portal system.	121 (BDC-3)	542, 302	F21(RS4)
4. Describe corpus callosum. Add a note to its role in cerebral asymmetry.	142	546	J09

Short Essays

1. Draw a neat labeled diagram to show the sulci, gyri, functional areas of the superolateral surface of the cerebrum.	127, 132	528	D13
2. Insula.	129	529	J19(RS3)
3. Sulci and gyri of superolateral surface of cerebrum.	129	529	J17(RS3)
4. Functional areas and blood supply of superolateral surface of cerebrum.	129	534	D18(RS3)
5. Lateral geniculate body.	119	541	D98
6. Caudate nucleus.	138	551	D10(RS2), D19(RS3), D99

Contd...

Contd...

	BDC Vol:4	IBSANT3	
7. Corpus callosum.	142	546	D08(RS2), D11(RS3), D13(RS3), J17(RS3), D01, D03
8. Internal capsule of brain.	143	547	D05(RS2), N20(RS3), J03, D06
Short Answers			
1. Calcarine sulcus.	131	530	D11(RS3), D12(RS3), J02
2. Paracentral lobule—parts of the body controlled.	131	530	D19(RS3), J14
3. Broca's motor speech area.	134	534	D12(RS3), J02
4. Sensory speech area in the cerebrum.	135	—	D12
5. Speech areas of brain.	147	534	J15(RS3)
6. Components of basal ganglia.	138	551	D10
7. Name white fibers of cerebrum.	141	545	J11
8. Association fibers of cerebrum.	141	545	D16
9. Mention commissural fibers of cerebral hemisphere.	141	545	D01, J08
10. Corpus callosum (parts).	142	546	D18(RS3), J15
11. Parts of internal capsule.	144	547	D05

CHAPTER 93: THIRD VENTRICLE, LATERAL VENTRICLE AND LIMBIC SYSTEM

Short Essays

1. Third ventricle.	123	559	D17(RS3), J05
2. Describe the boundaries of the lateral ventricle.	123	557	J13
3. Inferior horn of lateral ventricle.	150	559	J19(RS3)

Contd...

Contd...

	BDC Vol:4	IBSANT3	
Short Answers			
1. Recesses of third ventricle.	123	560	N20(RS3)
2. Inferior horn of lateral ventricle.	150	559	D14
3. Papez circuit of recent memory.	155	—	D09

CHAPTER 94: SOME NEURAL PATHWAYS AND RETICULAR FORMATION

Short Answers			
1. What are gray and white rami communicants?	—	—	D13
2. Effects of upper motor neuron lesion.	159	484	D08

CHAPTER 95: BLOOD SUPPLY OF SPINAL CORD AND BRAIN

Long Essay			
1. Write diagram of circle of Willis and anterior cerebral artery and its branches. Name areas that anterior cerebral artery supplies.	165	577	J06(RS2)
Short Essays			
1. Choroid plexus.	—	558	D00
2. Spinal cord—blood supply.	162	459	J05(RS2), D12(RS3), D18(RS3)
3. Circle of Willis (circulus arteriosus).	165	577	J07(RS2), D09(RS2), J10(RS2), J11(RS2). D98
Short Answers			
1. Choroid plexus.	—	558	J14
2. What is subarachnoid hemorrhage? Mention one cause.	—	—	J06
3. Basilar artery (branches).	163	580	D10(RS2), J12(RS3), J15(RS3)
4. List any four functional areas of the cerebrum supplied by the middle cerebral artery.	165	582	J14

Contd...

ANATOMY

Contd...

	BDC Vol:4	IBSANT3	
5. Draw and label circle of Willis.	166	578	J15
6. Blood-brain barrier—components, functional importance.	167	589	F21(RS4)

	IBSEMB	KDSN	

SECTION 8: EMBRYOLOGY

CHAPTER 96: INTRODUCTION AND SOME PRELIMINARY CONSIDERATIONS

None.

CHAPTER 97: GENETICS AND MOLECULAR BIOLOGY IN EMBRYOLOGY

Short Essays

	IBSEMB	KDSN	
1. X chromosome.	—	—	J08(RS2)
2. Y chromosome.	—	—	D08(RS2)
3. Compare and contrast the features of autosomal dominant and autosomal recessive inheritance.	—	—	F21(RS4)
4. Meiosis.	—	12	J15
5. Non-disjunction and its consequences.	—	8	D11(RS3), D16
6. Gene.	8	5	D15(RS3)
7. Chromosome.	7	7	J06(RS2), D19(RS3)
8. Types/classification of chromosomes.	7	7	D13(RS3), D14
9. Karyotyping—principles and applications.	10	8	D08(RS2), J09(RS2), D15(RS3), D17(RS3), J98, J09, J13
10. Abnormalities of chromosome.	11	—	J12(RS3)
11. Numerical chromosomal anomalies.	11	—	J16(RS3)

Contd...

Contd...

	IBSEMB	KDSN	
12. Down's syndrome/trisomy 21 (causes and symptoms).	11	8	J13(RS3), J14(RS3), D16(RS3), N20(RS3), D99, D11, J14, D15
13. Trisomy 18.	11	8	J11
14. Turner's syndrome.	11	9	J10(RS2), J19(RS3), J10
15. Klinefelter's syndrome.	11	9	J05(RS2), D07(RS2), J15(RS3), J17(RS3), D18(RS3)
16. Autosomal dominant inheritance.	—	5	J10(RS2), D11(RS3), J18(RS3)
17. Sex-linked inheritance.	—	—	J99
18. Genetic counseling.	11	—	J21(RS4), D07(RS2)
Short Answers			
1. Ribonucleic acid (RNA).	—	—	J18(RS3)
2. X chromosome.	—	—	J12(RS3)
3. Y chromosome.	—	—	D98, J09
4. Anaphase lag.	—	—	D03
5. Robersonian translocation.	—	—	D18(RS3), D03
6. Aneuploidy.	—	—	D03
7. Chromosomal bandings.	—	—	D10
8. Write any three differences between mitosis and meiosis.	—	—	D02
9. Mendel's law of independent assortment with example.	—	—	D16(RS3), J17(RS3)
10. Genetic code	—	—	J10
11. Monosomy.	—	—	D05
12. Polyploidy.	—	4	J04

Contd...

Contd...

	IBSEMB	KDSN	
13. Recessive genes.	—	5	J00, D01, D02, J03
14. Genome.	—	5	J05(RS2)
15. What is Philadelphia chromosome?	—	8	D09
16. Meiotic non-disjunction—mechanism and consequences.	—	8	F21(RS4), D98, J01, J02, J03, D04, D05, J12, J13
17. Meiosis—stages, significance.	—	12	D05(RS2), D98, J07
18. Autosomes.	7	—	D06
19. Sex chromosomes.	7	—	D06(RS2)
20. Chromosome	7	7	D17(RS3), J10, J12
21. Define chromosome. Give the chromosome complement of normal male and female.	7	7	J00
22. Mention the types of chromosomes based on centromere position.	9	—	D16
23. What is the difference between metacentric, submetacentric and acrocentric chromosomes?	9	—	J03
24. Satellite bodies.	9	—	J04
25. List six acrocentric chromosomes.	10	—	J07
26. Name the chromosomes with satellite bodies.	10	—	D01
27. Karyotyping—diagnostic importance.	10	8	D98, J05, J12, D15
28. Lyon's hypothesis.	11	—	D19(RS3)
29. Ring chromosome.	—	—	D07
30. Mention any three structural abnormalities of chromosomes.	—	—	J00, J03, D09
31. Describe translocation of chromosomes.	—	4	J21(RS4), J04, D05
32. Simian palmar crease.	—	—	D05
33. Name any three syndromes having trisomy.	11	—	J04

Contd...

Contd...

	IBSEMB	KDSN	
34. Down's syndrome—karyotype and clinical feature.	11	8	D05(RS2), D09(RS2), D10(RS2), J98, D02, D03, D14
35. Trisomy.	11	8	J07(RS2)
36. Turner's syndrome—karyotype, phenotype, causes and clinical features.	11	9	D06(RS2), D19(RS3), D99, D00, J02, J04, J07, D07, J12, J13, J14
37. Klinefelter's syndrome—karyotype, phenotype and clinical feature.	11	9	D08(RS2), J06, D98, J99, D01, D03, D10, D12, J15
38. Mutation.	16	5	J07(RS2), J11(RS2)
39. What is pedigree analysis?	—	—	D12
40. Define genotype and phenotype.	—	5	D10(RS2), J00, J01, D04, D07, J08, D08
41. Name any four X-linked inheritances.	11	—	J13
42. Name any three autosomal dominant disorders.	11	5	D08
43. Autosomal dominance.	11	5	J00, J02, D10
44. Recessive trait.	11	5	D06
45. Name any four autosomal recessive disorders.	11	6	D07
46. Genetic counseling.	11	—	J99, D99
47. Mention the examples of X-linked recessive inheritance.	11	—	D09, D11
Multiple Choice Questions			
1. The number of X chromosomes in patient with Turner's syndrome are __________. a. 0 b. **1** c. 2 d. 3	11	9	J21(RS4)

Contd...

Contd...

	IBSEMB	KDSN	
CHAPTER 98: REPRODUCTIVE SYSTEM, GAMETOGENESIS, OVARIAN AND MENSTRUAL CYCLE			
Short Essays			
1. Spermatogenesis.	20	27	J10(RS2), J19(RS3), D16
2. Capacitation.	21	51	D11(RS3)
3. Oogenesis.	22	29	J09(RS2), D15(RS3)
4. Graafian follicle (formation).	23	31	J11, J13
Short Answers			
1. Name any three investigations for infertility.	—	—	D01
2. Draw and label the structure of a spermatozoon (longitudinal section).	19	25	J00, D08, J12, J15
3. Mention the chromosomal complement of spermatogonium and spermatozoa.	19	28	J02
4. Spermiogenesis (stages).	20	27	J07(RS2), D98, J03, J10, D13
5. Write diagrammatic representation of spermatocytogenesis.	21	—	J03
6. Capacitation.	21	51	D00
7. Write diagrammatic representation of stages in oogenesis.	22	30	D01
8. Graafian follicle (draw and label).	23	31	D08
9. Ovulation	24	35	J15(RS3)
10. Corpus luteum.	23	37	J10, D12
CHAPTER 99: FIRST WEEK OF DEVELOPMENT—STAGES OF EMBRYOLOGY/GESTATIONAL PERIOD			
Short Essays			
1. Fertilization and its effects.	35	49	J12(RS3), J11(RS2), J14(RS3), D19(RS3), D99

Contd...

Contd...

	IBSEMB	KDSN	
2. Cleavage and morula.	39	54	D15
3. Trophoblast.	40	54	J05(RS2)
4. Describe the process of formation of the blastocyst with the help of a neat labeled diagram.	40	54	J21(RS4), J11(RS2)
5. Implantation.	41	56, 75	D13(RS3), D17(RS3), J03
Short Answers			
1. Zygosis.	—	—	J03
2. Fertilization and its results.	35	52	D18(RS3), J19(RS3), J08, J13, J15, D15
3. What is the acrosome reaction?	37	51	D10
4. In vitro fertilization.	39	53	D07(RS2)
5. Morula.	39	54	J00, D00, J05
6. Blastocyst (neat, labeled diagram).	40	54	F21(RS4), D16(RS3), J01, D04, J06, J07, D07, D08, D14
7. Zona pellucida.	38	55	J02, J11
8. Mention any two types of implantation with examples.	41	81	J02
9. Decidua (name three layers).	44	81	J09, D09
10. Ectopic pregnancy.	43	85	D08(RS2)

CHAPTER 100: SECOND WEEK OF DEVELOPMENT—BILAMINAR GERM DISK FORMATION

Short Essays			
1. Chorionic villi—formation.	51	82	J18(RS3), D13
Short Answers			
1. Prochordal plate.	49	61	D01

Contd...

Contd...

	IBSEMB	KDSN	
2. Chorion—formation and fate.	51	61	D15(RS3)
3. Chorionic villi.	51	82	D05(RS2), J08(RS2), J11
4. Name the three types of villi with structural differences in a developing placenta.	51	82	J01, D04, D07
5. Tertiary chorionic villus (labeled diagram).	53	82	D03, D05

CHAPTER 101: THIRD WEEK OF DEVELOPMENT—GERMINAL PERIOD

Short Essays

1. Trilaminar germ disk.	60	60	D10
2. Primitive streak.	59	61	J16(RS3), J01, D01
3. Gastrulation.	60	62	D12(RS3)
4. Notochord—development, functions and fate.	60	66	D06(RS2), J08(RS2), J13(RS3), D14(RS3), J17(RS3), D18(RS3), D03, D05, D06
5. Explain the formation of intra-embryonic mesoderm and mention the subdivisions.	63	62	D12

Short Answers

1. Bilaminar germ disc.	59	59	J06(RS2)
2. Primitive streak (formation).	59	61	J07(RS2), D98, J07, J09, D13
3. Explain the process of gastrulation.	60	62	J21(RS4)
4. Give the structure arising from primitive streak.	60	62	D11
5. Hensen's node.	60	66	N20(RS3)
6. Name the derivatives of notochord.	62	66	J98, J99, J03
7. Division and derivatives of intraembryonic mesoderm.	63	62	J14(RS3), J12

Contd...

Contd...

	IBSEMB	KDSN	
CHAPTER 102: EMBRYONIC PERIOD OF DEVELOPMENT			
Short Essays			
1. Mesodermal somites.	68	63	D07(RS2)
2. Septum transversum.	72	166	J01
Short Answers			
1. Cloacal membrane.	73	62	J00
2. What is septum transversum and name the structure derived from it.	72	166	J18(RS3), J12
CHAPTER 103: FETAL PERIOD OF DEVELOPMENT			
Short Essays			
1. Prenatal diagnosis—purpose and methods.	80	96	J09(RS2), D12
2. Amniocentesis.	80	95	D14(RS3)
Short Answers			
1. Name two teratogens.	80	—	J06
2. Prenatal diagnosis (different types, name two techniques).	80	96	J12(RS3), J01, D01, D04, D08, D09, J14
CHAPTER 104: PLACENTA, FETAL MEMBRANE AND TWINNING			
Short Essays			
1. Amnion.	85	61	D06(RS2)
2. Yolk sac.	86	59, 66	D08(RS2), J09
3. Describe the development of umbilical cord. Explain why the umbilical arteries carry deoxygenated blood and umbilical veins carry oxygenated blood.	87	90	F21(RS4)
4. Umbilical cord—formation, contents.	87	90	J04
Short Answers			
1. Placenta previa.	89	85	J10(RS2)
2. What are the differences between fetal and maternal side of the placenta?	90	—	J13

Contd...

ANATOMY

Contd...

	IBSEMB	KDSN	
3. Placental barrier.	92	83	D11(RS3), J04, J08
4. Functions of placenta.	92	83	D11(RS3), D98, J15
5. Name the fetal membranes.	85	—	D15
6. Amniotic fluids—formation and functions.	85	94	J99, J06
7. Yolk sac.	86	59, 66	J99, J07, D07, J08
8. Vitellointestinal (viteline) duct.	88	68	J17(RS3), D12
9. Umbilical cord—contents.	88	90	J08(RS2), N20(RS3), J99, D06
10. Monozygotic twins.	95	349	D07(RS2)

CHAPTER 105: FORMATION OF TISSUES OF THE BODY

Short Answers

1. Name any four derivatives of endoderm.	101	—	D00, J04
2. Mention any four derivatives of mesoderm.	101	—	D02
3. Paraxial mesoderm and its derivatives.	101	63	D98, D08, D13

CHAPTER 106: INTEGUMENTARY SYSTEM (SKIN AND ITS APPENDAGES, MAMMARY GLAND)

None

CHAPTER 107: PHARYNGEAL ARCHES

Short Essays

1. First pharyngeal arch (derivatives, nerve of arch).	128	98	D05(RS2), D09(RS2), J14(RS3), D02, J08, J15
2. Second pharyngeal arch (derivatives).	128	102	D11(RS3), D10
3. Tubotympanic recess.	131	106	J05

Contd...

Contd...

	IBSEMB	KDSN	
4. Development of thyroid gland—description with labeled diagram and common congenital anomalies.	133	138	D15(RS3), J06, D09, J10
5. Microscopic structure and development of thyroid gland.	133	138	D06
Short Answers			
1. Second pharyngeal arch and its derivatives.	128	102	J08(RS2), J19(RS3)
2. Derivatives of 1st pharyngeal arch, pouch and cleft.	128, 131	102, 106	D16(RS3)
3. Meckel's cartilage and its fate.	128	102	D08(RS2), D09(RS2)
4. Derivatives of first pharyngeal/brachial arch.	128	98	J15(RS3), D19(RS3)
5. Mention the mesodermal (skeletal) derivatives of hyoid (2nd branchial) arch.	129	102	J98, D99
6. Development of the styloid process of the temporal bone.	129	101	D05
7. Mention the derivatives of third branchial arch.	129	101	J17(RS3)
8. Development of hyoid bone.	129	101	J12(RS3), J01, D04
9. Fate of ectodermal clefts.	130	106	D07(RS2)
10. Name the muscles of first pharyngeal arch.	130	102	D14
11. Derivatives of 1st pharyngeal pouch.	131	106	J10(RS2), D07
12. Derivatives of 3rd pharyngeal pouch.	131	107	D10(RS2)
13. Development of palatine tonsil	132	107	J06(RS2)
14. Mention the development of thymus.	132	107	J98, J10, D12
15. Development of the parathyroid glands.	132	143	D09(RS2), D10(RS2), J99
16. Thyroid gland development.	133	138	J15
17. Thyroglossal duct.	133	138	D12(RS3)

Contd...

ANATOMY

Contd...

	IBSEMB	KDSN	

CHAPTER 108: SKELETAL SYSTEM AND MUSCULAR SYSTEM

Short Essay

	IBSEMB	KDSN	
1. Somite.	138	63	J11(RS2), D16(RS3), J98, D09

Short Answers

	IBSEMB	KDSN	
1. Clinodactyly.	—	—	D06
2. Webbed neck.	—	—	D06
3. Somite	138	63	J06(RS2)
4. Give the parts of body somites.	138	63	D11
5. Sclerotome.	138	63	D11
6. Dermatome.	138	21	J12(RS3), D13(RS3), D14(RS3), J07, J11
7. Myotome.	138	21	J16(RS3)

CHAPTER 109: FACE, NOSE AND PALATE

Short Essays

	IBSEMB	KDSN	
1. Development of the face—description with labeled diagram and its anomalies.	150	144	D05
2. Facial clefts.	157	149	J05
3. Development of palate.	156	152	J17(RS3)

Short Answers

	IBSEMB	KDSN	
1. Development of face.	150	144	D08(RS2)
2. Cleft lip.	153	148	D10(RS2)

CHAPTER 110: ALIMENTARY SYSTEM I: MOUTH, PHARYNX AND RELATED STRUCTURES

Short Essays

	IBSEMB	KDSN	
1. Development of tongue and common congenital anomalies.	165	133	D07(RS2), D10(RS2), J19(RS3), D00, J02, D04, D10, D14

Contd...

ANATOMY

Contd...

	IBSEMB	KDSN	
2. Tongue—lymphatic drainage and development.	165	133	J11(RS2)
3. Tongue—development and nerve supply.	165	133	D16(RS3)
4. Hypobranchial eminence.	166	133	J12(RS3)
Short Answers			
1. Development of tongue.	165	133	J07(RS2), J16(RS3)
2. Name three developmental anomalies of the tongue	167	135	J21(RS4)

CHAPTER 111: ALIMENTARY SYSTEM II: GASTROINTESTINAL TRACT

Short Essays			
1. Name the parts derived from the foregut, midgut and hindgut.	174	171	D12
2. Developmental derivatives of midgut.	174	171	J11(RS2), J18(RS3)
3. Development of rectum and anal canal.	181	191	J09(RS2)
4. Development of anal canal and anomalies.	181	191	J12
5. Rotation of gut (midgut).	183	195	D08(RS2), J15(RS3), J14, D14
6. Discuss the congenital anomalies associated with umbilicus.	180	92	J14
Short Answers			
1. What is allantois and what is its fate after birth?	—	—	D15
2. Derivatives of foregut.	174	171	J16(RS3), D17(RS3), J04, D08, J14, J15, D16
3. Derivatives of midgut.	174	171	J08(RS2), D09(RS2), D11(RS3), D14(RS3), J99, J01, J02, J03, D04, D07, J08

Contd...

Contd...

	IBSEMB	KDSN	
4. Derivatives of hindgut.	174	171	J10(RS2), D10(RS2), J00, D00, D03
5. Ventral mesogastrium and its derivatives.	175	177	J06(RS2), J98, D99, J00, D01, J06, J11
6. Name the structures developing in the ventral and dorsal mesogastrium.	175	177	D13
7. Derivatives of the dorsal mesogastrium.	175	177	D02
8. Cecal bud.	172	189	D05
9. Development of cecum.	172	189	D02
10. Development of vermiform appendix.	172	189	D11(RS3), D98
11. How does transverse colon develop?	183	190	J13
12. Development of rectum and anal canal.	183	191	J11(RS2)
13. What are the sources of development of anal canal?	183	191	J13, D15
14. Hirschsprung's disease or congenital megacolon.	181	193	J09
15. Imperforate anus.	181	195	D06
16. What are the complications of the persistent vitelline duct?	181	199	D13
17. Omphalocele.	181	198	J02
18. Situs inversus.	181	202	D06

CHAPTER 112: LIVER AND BILIARY APPARATUS; PANCREAS AND SPLEEN

Short Essays

1. Blood supply and development of pancreas.	192	186	D14

Contd...

ANATOMY

Contd...

	IBSEMB	KDSN	
2. Development of pancreas and congenital anomalies.	192	186	J06(RS2), D07(RS2), J09(RS2), J17(RS3), D17(RS3), D18(RS3), J19(RS3), J00, D07, D09, D11, D16
3. Development of spleen.	195	179	J07(RS2), D11(RS3)
Short Answers			
1. Development of extrahepatic biliary system.	191	183	J17(RS3)
2. Development of gallbladder.	191	183	J02
3. Development of pancreas.	192	186	J16(RS3), D98, D00, D08, J13
4. Ventral pancreatic bud.	192	186	D05
5. Parts of pancreas developed from dorsal pancreatic bud.	194	186	J03
6. Annular pancreas.	195	188	J07(RS2)
7. Development of spleen.	195	179	D17(RS3), D19(RS3), D98, J10

CHAPTER 113: BODY CAVITIES, DIAPHRAGM AND RESPIRATORY SYSTEM

Long Essay			
1. Describe the development of lung. Add a note on its congenital anomalies.	268, 214	160	J14(RS3)
Short Essay			
1. Development and developmental anomalies of diaphragm.	206	166	D15
Short Answers			
1. Development of diaphragm.	206	166	J02

Contd...

ANATOMY

Contd...

	IBSEMB	KDSN	
2. Tracheoesophageal fistula—embryological basis.	215	172	F21(RS4)
3. Maturation of lung.	216	160	J04

CHAPTER 114: CARDIOVASCULAR SYSTEM

Short Essays

1. Interatrial septum—development, congenital anomalies, applied anatomy.	223	207	J12(RS3), D16(RS3), J02, D04, J08, J09, J10
2. Development of right atrium.	224	208	J09(RS2)
3. Fallot's tetralogy.	227	220	D14
4. Ligamentum arteriosum.	234	223	D10(RS2), J01, J15
5. Arch of aorta—development, and mention one congenital anomaly of it.	234	224	J16(RS3), J06
6. Development of portal vein.	303	237	J05(RS2), J10(RS2)

Short Answers

1. Development of interatrial septum.	223	207	J13(RS3)
2. Septum spurium.	223	208	D14(RS3)
3. Septum secundum.	249	207	J16(RS3)
4. Fate of sinus venosus.	231	208	J15(RS3), D02
5. Fossa ovalis in the fetus.	224	208	D15
6. Spiral septum.	225	210	D13(RS3), D17(RS3)
7. Name three sources of development of interventricular septum.	225	213	J21(RS4), J99
8. Probe patency test.	227	—	J04
9. Fallot's tetralogy (anatomical defect).	227	220	J09(RS2), D01, D03, D10
10. What is ductus arteriosus? Give its fate.	251	223	J05(RS2), D07, D09, D15

Contd...

ANATOMY

Contd...

	IBSEMB	KDSN	
11. What is ligamentum arteriosum? Mention its embryological significance.	234	223	J98, D12
12. Development of arch of aorta.	234	224	D11(RS3), J10
13. Ductus venosus (functions and fate).	249	237	D03, J07
14. Left common cardinal vein (structures developed).	244	239	D09
15. Subcardinal veins.	245	244	J02
16. Shunts in fetal circulation and their fate after birth.	249	249	J14(RS3)
17. Name any two important changes in the fetal circulation soon after birth.	250	—	D02
Multiple Choice Questions			
1. Ligamentum teres hepatis is remnant of _______. a. Umbilical arteries b. **Left umbilical vein** c. Ductus venosus d. Ductus arteriosus	241	239	J21(RS4)

CHAPTER 115: UROGENITAL SYSTEM

Short Essays			
1. Cloaca.	259	191	D12(RS3), J17(RS3)
2. Development of kidney and its anomalies.	259	256	D17(RS3), J99
3. Describe the development of the kidney. Explain the embryological basis of congenital polycystic kidney.	259, 262	256, 264	F21(RS4)
4. Mesonephric duct—development and derivatives.	259, 260	258	D05(RS2), D99, J05, J10, D13
5. Describe the ascent of the kidney and associated congenital anomalies.	261	260	D15
6. Development and anomalies of urinary bladder.	262	268	J05(RS2), D07(RS2), D16(RS3), D09

Contd...

ANATOMY

Contd...

	IBSEMB	KDSN	
7. Paramesonephric duct and its fate in both sexes.	266	274, 278	D08(RS2), J12(RS3), D16(RS3), N20(RS3), J11, D11, J15
8. Development of uterus and its anomalies.	266	274	J14(RS3), D19(RS3), J98
9. Development of external genital organs.	269	279	J13(RS3)
10. Testis—development, developmental anomalies and its descent.	272	283	D13(RS3), D15(RS3), J16(RS3)
11. Describe the development of the ovary.	278	291	J21(RS4)
Short Answers			
1. Streak gonads.	—	—	D06
2. Holonephros.	—	—	J12
3. Ectodermal cloaca.	—	—	J03
4. Name any four derivatives of endodermal cloaca.	—	191	D06, J09
5. Prostatic utricle (development).	—	272	D06, J09
6. Gartner's duct.	—	295	D10
7. Subdivisions of cloaca.	259	170	J08
8. Cloaca.	259	191	J12(RS3)
9. Name the parts of the kidney derived from metanephric blastema and mesonephric duct.	259	259	J13
10. Ureteric bud.	259	266	J11
11. Mesonephric duct—formation and fate.	262	258	J14(RS3)
12. Metanephric blastema.	262	—	J04
13. Name derivatives of ureteric bud.	260	256	J00
14. Name any four development anomalies of kidneys.	261	261	J00, D02
15. Polycystic kidney.	262	264	D06, D07
16. Formation and fate of vesicourethral canal.	259	265	D14(RS3)

Contd...

Contd...

	IBSEMB	KDSN	
17. Development of urinary bladder.	259	268	D10
18. Development of trigone of bladder.	263	268	D05, J08
19. Urachus and its remnants.	263	268	J00
20. What is the fate of the allantois?	263	268	J14
21. Development of prostatic urethra.	265	270	D11
22. Describe the development of the prostate.	265	272	D02
23. Development of uterus.	266	274	D09(RS2)
24. Formation and fate of paramesonephric (Mullerian) duct.	266	274, 278	D13(RS3), D05
25. Anomalies of development of uterus.	267	276	D13(RS3)
26. Imperforate hymen.	267	278	J09
27. Derivatives of primordial germ cells.	272	—	J06
28. Hypospadias.	272	282	D09(RS2), D11(RS3), D07, J14
29. Epispadias.	272	282	D06
30. Processus vaginalis.	340	286	D15(RS3)
31. Anomalies of development of testis.	278	288	J14(RS3)
32. Name the derivatives of gubernaculum of ovary in females.	274	—	D08
33. Derivatives of mesonephric duct (in males/females).	274	258	J10(RS2), D10(RS2), D18(RS3), J98, D01, D03, J07, J08, D08, J12
34. Derivatives of paramesonephric duct (in females).	266	274	D06(RS2), D98, D02, J02, J05, J10

CHAPTER 116: NERVOUS SYSTEM

Short Essay

1. Describe the neural tube formation and associated anomalies of the neural tube.	283	65, 297	J15(RS3), J14

Contd...

Contd...

	IBSEMB	KDSN	
Short Answer			
1. Neural crest cells and its derivatives.	285	298	J09(RS2), D98, J99, D00, D05, D08

CHAPTER 117: ENDOCRINE GLANDS

Short Essays			
1. Histology and development of hypophysis cerebri.	306	338	J14(RS3)
2. Development of suprarenal gland.	307	341	D14(RS3)
3. Development and microscopic structure of suprarenal gland.	307	341	J08
Short Answers			
1. How hypophysis cerebri is developed.	306	338	J10(RS2), J98
2. Development of adrenal (suprarenal) gland.	307	341	J12(RS3), D11, D14

CHAPTER 118: DEVELOPMENT OF EYE

Short Answer			
1. Development of tympanic membrane.	319	321	J06

	IBSHST	DFIOR	

SECTION 9: HISTOLOGY

CHAPTER 119: LIGHT MICROSCOPY AND TISSUE PREPARATION

None

CHAPTER 120: CELL STRUCTURE

Short Essay			
1. Barr body (sex chromatin).	—	—	J07(RS2), N20(RS3)
Short Answers			
1. Mitochondria.	12	15	D09(RS2), J99, D00, D02

Contd...

Contd...

	IBSHST	DFIOR	
2. Golgi apparatus/body.	13	16	J99, J02
3. Centrioles.	15	18	J03, J11
4. Barr body (sex chromatin).	—	—	J05(RS2), J09(RS2), D10(RS2), J11(RS2), D12(RS3), J98, D99, J00, D02, D05, J06, J08, D11, D14, J15

CHAPTER 121: EPITHELIA AND GLANDS

Short Essays

1. Draw a neat labeled diagram of transitional epithelium (urothelium). Mention all the regions in the body where transitional epithelium is present.	34	53	J21(RS4), J04, D11
2. Compare and contrast the light microscopic features of serous and mucous acini.	37	60	F21(RS4)

Short Answers

1. Simple squamous epithelium.	21	48	J11
2. Draw and label the microscopic structure of pseudostratified columnar ciliated epithelium.	22	53	D11
3. Stratified squamous epithelium.	22	52	D08(RS2)
4. Draw a labeled diagram of the stratified squamous keratinized epithelium.	23	55	D13
5. Name the three sites of stratified squamous nonkeratinized epithelium.	34	56	J08
6. Transitional epithelium (urothelium).	34	55	J09(RS2), J10(RS2), D18(RS3), D98, J09
7. Name the types of cells present in the transitional epithelium and mention their functions.	34	53	J13

Contd...

Contd...

	IBSHST	DFIOR	
8. Draw a labeled diagram of transitional epithelium (urothelium).	35	53	J01, D04, D07
9. Basement membrane.	35	47	J99
10. Microvilli.	27	19	J98, D14
11. Brush border.	27	353	J11
12. Classify glands according to mode of secretion with one example each.	36	60	J14(RS3)
13. Mucus acinous.	37	60	J11

CHAPTER 122: GENERAL CONNECTIVE TISSUE

None

CHAPTER 123: CARTILAGE

Short Essays

1. Microscopic anatomy of the hyaline cartilage.	58	121	J15(RS3), D16(RS3), J19(RS3), J02, D04, D12
2. Microscopic structure of elastic cartilage.	58	123	J12(RS3), J16(RS3), D08(RS2), D16

Short Answers

1. Perichondrium.	56	119	J17(RS3)
2. Examples of the hyaline cartilage in the body.	58	118	D98, D03
3. Articular cartilage—structure.	58	121	D07
4. Labeled diagram of hyaline cartilage.	58	121	J05(RS2), J06, J12
5. Give any four features of hyaline cartilage.	58	121	D00
6. Elastic cartilage (examples).	60	118	J99, J04
7. Neat labeled diagram of microstructure of elastic cartilage.	61	123	D13
8. Histology of (white) fibrocartilage (draw and label).	61	124	J07, D11

Contd...

Contd...

	IBSHST	DFIOR	
9. Differences between hyaline and elastic cartilage.	63	118	D12

CHAPTER 124: BONE

Short Essays

1. Haversian system.	76	132	D09
2. Histology of compact bone.	71	144	N20(RS3)
3. Microscopic structure of transverse section of compact bone (labeled diagram, distinguishing features).	76	144	J18(RS3), J06, J13

Short Answers

1. Name three types of cells in the bone and their locations.	66	133	J01, D04
2. Osteon.	76	132	J19(RS3)
3. Draw a labeled diagram of Haversian system.	70	144	D00
4. Draw a labeled diagram of the microscopic structure of compact bone.	71	144	J08(RS2), D13(RS3), J14(RS3), J02

CHAPTER 125: MUSCULAR TISSUE

Short Essays

1. Microscopic structure of skeletal muscle.	84, 82	156	D15
2. Microscopic structure of cardiac muscle.	89	164	J11(RS2)

Short Answers

1. Sarcomere.	86	154	D16(RS3), J19(RS3), D98
2. Draw and label microscopic structure of sarcomere.	86	155	J12
3. Any three differences between histology of skeletal and cardiac muscle.	88	—	J08
4. Histology of cardiac muscle.	93	164	J12(RS3), N20(RS3), J07
5. Intercalated disc.	89	163	D98

Contd...

Contd...

	IBSHST	DFIOR	
CHAPTER 126: LYMPATHICS AND LYMPHOID TISSUE			
Short Essays			
1. Microscopic structure of lymph node (labeled diagram, specific distinguishing features).	99	253	J05(RS2), J17(RS3), D18(RS3), J98, D99, D01, J05, D05, D06
2. Microscopic structure of palatine tonsil (neat labeled diagram).	108	265	D07(RS2), D08(RS2), J18(RS3), D09, D13
Short Answers			
1. Role of colchicine in lymphocyte culture.	—	—	D10
2. Mention two histological differences between spleen and tonsil.	100	—	D05
3. Microscopic structure of lymph node. (draw a neat labeled diagram).	99	253	J07(RS2), D11(RS3), J13(RS3), D14(RS3), J00, J08, D15
4. Microscopic structure of spleen (draw and label).	101	262	D16(RS3), D04, D10
5. White pulp of spleen.	101	264	D08, D11
6. Red pulp.	100	264	J04
7. Hassel's corpuscles (location and embryological significance).	104	259	J98, J07, D10
8. Labeled diagram of the microscopic structure of thymus.	105	259	D17(RS3), J19(RS3), D02, J12, J15
9. Draw and label microscopic structure of palatine tonsil.	108	265	J10(RS2), J16(RS3)
CHAPTER 127: NERVOUS SYSTEM			
Short Essays			
1. Microscopic anatomy of transverse section of peripheral nerve.	119	211	D12(RS3)
2. Draw and label the microstructure of the sensory ganglion.	121	214	J14

Contd...

Contd...

	IBSHST	DFIOR	
3. Microscopic anatomy of sympathetic ganglion.	123	215	D10
Short Answers			
1. Nissl's substance.	112	188	J00, D00, D01
2. Dorsal root ganglion.	123	214	D12
3. List four typical microscopic anatomical features of the dorsal root ganglion.	123	214	J07
4. Draw and label microscopic structure of spinal ganglion.	123	214	D07(RS2)
5. Three differences between structure of spinal ganglion and autonomic ganglion.	122	—	D07

CHAPTER 128: CARDIOVASCULAR SYSTEM

Short Essay			
1. Muscular artery—microscopic anatomy.	129	232	D06(RS2)
Short Answers			
1. Name the layers found in the wall of a vessel.	125	224	D10
2. Draw and label microscopic structure of elastic artery (large artery).	130	234	D08(RS2), J09(RS2), D18(RS3)
3. Give three differences in the structure of elastic artery and muscular artery.	129	—	D08
4. Labeled diagram of histology of muscular artery (medium-sized artery).	130	232	D09(RS2), D03, J07, J12, D15

CHAPTER 129: SKIN AND ITS APPENDAGES

Short Essays			
1. Microscopic structure of thin skin (labeled diagram) difference from the thick skin.	140	277	J03

Contd...

Contd...

	IBSHST	DFIOR	
2. Draw and label microscopic structure of thick skin.	139	282	D11(RS3)
Short Answer			
1. Myoepitheliocytes.	146	281	D10(RS2)

CHAPTER 130: SALIVARY GLAND

Short Essays			
1. Histology of parotid gland.	154	312	J10(RS2)
2. Microscopic structure of submandibular salivary gland.	155	314	D11(RS3)
Short Answers			
1. Labeled diagram of microscopic structure of serous salivary glands (parotid gland).	156	313	D16(RS3), D01, D14
2. Draw and label microscopic structure of mixed salivary gland.	155	314	J12

CHAPTER 131: PLACENTA AND UMBILICAL CORD

Short Essay			
1. Microscopic structure of the placenta.	162	555	J09(RS2)
Short Answers			
1. Microscopic structure of placenta (labeled diagram only).	162	555	J03
2. Labeled diagram of the microscopic structure of umbilical cord.	165	—	D07(RS2), J10(RS2)

CHAPTER 132: RESPIRATORY SYSTEM

Short Essays			
1. Describe the microscopic structure of trachea.	173	410	J14(RS3), D17(RS3)
2. Microscopic anatomy of lung (correlate with its function).	174	412	J21(RS4), D05(RS2), D13(RS3), D14(RS3)

Contd...

Contd...

	IBSHST	DFIOR	
Short Answers			
1. Microscopic structure of trachea.	173	410	J06(RS2), J09
2. Microscopic appearance of lung (only labeled diagram).	174	412	J02

CHAPTER 133: DIGESTIVE SYSTEM: ORAL CAVITY AND RELATED STRUCTURES

Short Essay			
1. Microscopic anatomy of tongue.	185	301	J13(RS3)
Short Answers			
1. Circumvallate papillae.	185	302	J11
2. Microscopic structure of tongue.	185	301	J12(RS3)
3. Microscopic appearance of lingual papillae (only labeled diagram).	185	303	D02
4. Draw and label taste bud.	188	304	J08(RS2)

CHAPTER 134: DIGESTIVE SYSTEM: GENERAL PLAN OF GASTROINTESTINAL TRACT, STOMACH AND INTESTINES

Short Essays			
1. Microscopic anatomy of fundus of stomach.	195	335	J19(RS3)
2. Microscopic structure of duodenum. .	210	355	J07(RS2), D07(RS2), D13(RS3), D18(RS3), J98, J10, D10
3. Microscopic structure of jejunum.	202	358	J05
4. Microscopic structure (histology) of ileum (draw and label).	203	361	J08(RS2), D11, D16
5. Microscopic structure of the vermiform appendix.	209	370	J05(RS2), J10(RS2), J18(RS3), D13, D14
Short Answers			
1. Plicae circulares.	—	353	D15(RS3)
2. Muscularis mucosa and its functions.	191	325	J00

Contd...

ANATOMY

Contd...

	IBSHST	DFIOR	
3. Esophageal glands.	192	326	J03
4. Fundic glands of stomach.	195	336	J00, D02
5. Histology of fundic part of stomach.	195	335	D07(RS2), J12(RS3), D05
6. Diagram of histology of pyloric end of stomach.	196	343	D03
7. Name the cells present in fundic part of stomach and give their secretion.	197	336	D07
8. Duodenal glands of Brunner.	200	354	J02, J04
9. Give any three differences in the structure of duodenum and jejunum	200	355	D08
10. Draw and label microscopic structure of duodenum.	201	355	D08(RS2), D09
11. Neat labeled diagram of microscopic structure of jejunum.	202	358	J01, D04, D06
12. Microscopic structure of ileum.	203	361	J11(RS2), D98, D03
13. Intestinal glands.	204	353	D15(RS3)
14. Crypts of Lieberkuhn.	204	353	D01
15. Goblet cell.	204	354	J15
16. Paneth cells—location, structure and functions.	205	354	J21(RS4)
17. Peyer's patches.	204	354	J00, J03, J11
18. Histological structure of vermiform appendix (only labeled diagram).	209	370	J09(RS2), D19(RS3), J03, J07, J12

CHAPTER 135: HEPATOBILIARY SYSTEM AND PANCREAS

Short Essays

1. Microscopic structure of liver (draw and label).	215	383	D05(RS2), D08(RS2), D10(RS2), J15(RS3), D17(RS3), J08, J13, J15
2. Gallbladder—microscopic structure and applied anatomy.	220	394	D09

Contd...

Contd...

	IBSHST	DFIOR	
3. Microscopic structure of pancreas.	223	389	J08(RS2), J10(RS2), D16(RS3), D19(RS3)
Short Answers			
1. Differentiate hepatic lobule from portal lobule.	—	380	J99
2. Draw and label classical lobule of liver.	215	381	D07
3. Portal triad (constituents).	215	380	J11
4. Neat labeled diagram of histological structure of liver.	218	383	D11(RS3), D00, J03
5. Portal lobule.	216	380	J12
6. Histology of gallbladder.	220	394	J09(RS2), D06, D10
7. Microscopic structure of pancreas (neat labeled diagram).	223	389	D14(RS3), D98, J04, J05, D05
8. Cells of islets of Langerhans.	224	390	N20(RS3), J14, J15
Multiple Choice Questions			
1. The cells of liver are the primary storehouse of vitamin A _________. a. Hepatocytes b. Kupffer cells c. Endothelial cells d. **Ito cells**	220	381	J21(RS4)
CHAPTER 136: URINARY SYSTEM			
Short Essays			
1. Microscopic structure of kidney (draw and label).	229	432	J05(RS2), J12(RS3), D12(RS3), D14(RS3), J17(RS3), N20(RS3), D15
2. Microscopic structure of ureter.	238	446	J09
3. Microscopic anatomy of urinary bladder (draw and label).	240	448	J16(RS3), D12

Contd...

Contd...

	IBSHST	DFIOR	
Short Answers			
1. Diagram showing parts of nephron (name the parts).	229	—	J02, J14
2. Diagram of histology of kidney.	229	432	J04, J06
3. Renal corpuscle (Malpighian corpuscle).	230	438	D98, J11
4. What are podocytes? Mention its functions.	230	—	J99
5. Microscopic structure of cortex of kidney.	229	433	J19(RS3)
6. Mention the lining epithelium of loop of Henle. What is its functional significance?	233	434	J98
7. Histology of medulla of kidney.	231	443	D06
8. Juxtaglomerular apparatus.	231	437	D02
9. Microstructure of ureter.	238	446	D05(RS2), J08(RS2), D10(RS2), J11(RS2), D99, J01, J03, D05, J06, D08
10. Diagram of histology of urinary bladder.	240	448	D08(RS2), D01, D03

CHAPTER 137: CENTRAL NERVOUS SYSTEM: SPINAL CORD, CEREBELLAR CORTEX AND CEREBRAL CORTEX

Short Essays			
1. Describe the microscopic structure of cerebrum.	248	192	J14(RS3)
2. Microscopic anatomy of cerebellum.	251	194	D15(RS3), D15
Short Answers			
1. Name the layers of the cerebral cortex.	248	192	D10
2. Draw a labeled diagram of microscopic structure of cerebellar cortex.	251	194	J10

Contd...

Contd...

	IBSHST	DFIOR	
CHAPTER 138: MALE REPRODUCTIVE SYSTEM			
Short Essays			
1. Microscopic structure of testis (draw and label).	257	493	D07(RS2), J13
2. Microscopic structure of epididymis	264	500	J11
3. Microscopic structure of vas deferens.	266	501	D08(RS2)
4. Histology of the prostate with a neat labeled diagram.	269	508	J14
Short Answers			
1. Microscopic appearance of testis (only labeled diagram).	257	493	D11(RS3), J12(RS3), D17(RS3), D02
2. Sertoli cells—structure and functions.	258	492	F21(RS4), J02, D12
3. Interstitial cells of Leydig.	258	489	D03
4. Microscopic structure of epididymis (draw and label).	264	500	D09(RS2), D18(RS3), D06
5. Mention two histological features of epididymis.	264	500	D99
6. Vas deferens—microscopy (only labeled diagram).	266	501	J06(RS2), J08(RS2), N20(RS3), D98
7. Corpora amylacea.	269	—	D03
8. Light microscopic structure of prostate gland (neat labeled diagram).	269	508	J06(RS2), J08(RS2), N20(RS3), D98
CHAPTER 139: FEMALE REPRODUCTIVE SYSTEM			
Short Essays			
1. Microscopic structure of ovary.	275	524	J06(RS2), D09(RS2), D11(RS3), J13(RS3), J14(RS3), D15(RS3), D99, D12, D13

Contd...

Contd...

	IBSHST	DFIOR	
2. Microscopic anatomy of the uterine tube (Fallopian tube)—draw and label.	281	533	D15
3. Microscopic structure of uterus (draw and label).	283	536	J07(RS2), D16
Short Answers			
1. Microscopic structure of ovary (draw and label).	275	524	J18(RS3), D98
2. Draw and label microscopic structure of Graafian follicle.	277	527	J10(RS2)
3. Corpus luteum (draw and label).	278	530	J00
4. Microscopic structure of fallopian tube (draw and label).	283	533	J12(RS3), D15(RS3), J17(RS3), D00, J02, D06, D07, J12
5. Endometrium.	280	522	J17(RS3)
6. Draw a neat labeled diagram of microscopic anatomy of uterus.	283	536	D13(RS3)
7. Microscopic appearance of endometrium in secretory phase (only labeled diagram).	283	537	D01

CHAPTER 140: ENDOCRINE SYSTEM

Short Essays			
1. Microscopic structure of pituitary gland.	297	463	D09(RS2), D19(RS3), D02
2. Histology and development of hypophysis cerebri.	297	463	J14(RS3)
3. Microscopic structure and development of thyroid gland.	303	473	D06
4. Microscopic structure (histology) of thyroid gland.	303	473	J07(RS2), J08(RS2), D10
5. Development and microscopic structure of suprarenal gland.	306	478	J08

Contd...

Contd...

	IBSHST	DFIOR	
6. Microscopic structure of the suprarenal gland.	306	478	D06(RS2), D11(RS3), J99, D10
7 Correlate the microstructure and functions of the adrenal cortex.	306	472	F21(RS4)
Short Answers			
1. What are the secretions from the basophilic cells of the pituitary gland?	296	462	J14
2. Microscopic appearance of hypophysis cerebri (only labeled diagram).	297	463	D01
3. Draw a labeled diagram of histology of a thyroid follicle.	303	474	D05
4. Describe the histological appearance of thyroid follicles in different stages of activity.	303	—	F21(RS4)
5. Microscopic structure of suprarenal gland (draw and label).	306	478	N20(RS3), J02, D05

CHAPTER 141: SPECIAL SENSES: EYE

Short Essay

1. Describe the microscopic structure of cornea.	315	573	D16(RS3)

Short Answer

1. Microscopic appearance of cornea (only labeled diagram).	315	573	D19(RS3), D02

CHAPTER 142: SPECIAL SENSES: EAR

None

2

PHYSIOLOGY

REFERENCES

1. GK Pal **(GKPAL)**: Comprehensive Textbook of Medical Physiology—Two volumes (3rd Edition Reprint), Jaypee Brothers Medical Publishers (P) Ltd., New Delhi, ₹ 1850/-
2. K Sembulingam **(SEMBU)**: Essentials of Medical Physiology (10th Edition), Jaypee Brothers Medical Publishers (P) Ltd., New Delhi ₹ 2095/-

Curriculum

	GKPAL	SEMBU	

SECTION 1: GENERAL PHYSIOLOGY

CHAPTER 1: DEFINING THE ROLE OF PHYSIOLOGY IN MODERN MEDICINE

None

CHAPTER 2: FUNCTIONAL ORGANIZATION OF HUMAN BODY

None

CHAPTER 3: PRINCIPLES OF HOMEOSTASIS

Short Essays

Question	GKPAL	SEMBU	
1. Explain feedback regulation with suitable examples.	10,11	41	F21(RS4)
2. Explain the role of 'positive feedback' regulation in endocrinology with one example.	11	41	D05(RS2), D13(RS3), J19(RS3)
3. What are negative feedback loops?	10	41	D09(RS2), J13(RS3)

Short Answers

Question	GKPAL	SEMBU	
1. Define "homeostasis" and "hemostasis".	9, 180	39, 113	D98
2. Homeostasis (define and give one example).	9	39	J13(RS3), D05
3. What is homeostasis? Describe positive feedback mechanism with suitable examples.	9,11	39, 41	D07
4. Give examples for 'negative feedback' and 'positive feedback' mechanisms in the body.	10	41	D12
5. Explain the positive feedback—mechanism of hormonal regulation with a suitable example.	11	41	D10(RS2), J02
6. Explain with the help of examples "negative feedback" mechanism of hormonal regulation.	10	41	J00

Contd...

Contd...

	GKPAL	SEMBU	
CHAPTER 4: CELLULAR ORGANIZATION AND INTERCELLULAR CONNECTIONS			
Short Essay			
1. Intercellular connections (cell junctions).	25	23	D09(RS2), D11(RS3), J17(RS3), D18(RS3)
Short Answers			
1. Enumerate various structures present in a cell (cell organelles). Give their functions.	14	4	D07
2. Structure of cell with a neat diagram.	14	4	J00
3. Mention the functions of proteins in cell membrane.	16	5	J21(RS4)
4. List the functions of cell membrane.	17	5	J13
5. Outline the structure of mitochondria and its function.	17	10,11	D15
6. Write the functions of 'endoplasmic reticulum.	19	7	D13
7. Mention the functions of (a) Mitochondria; (b) Golgi apparatus.	17,19	7	D09
8. Suicidal bags of a cell.	20	9	D16(RS3)
9. Mention the functions of (a) Ribosomes; (b) Lysosomes.	21, 20	9,11	D02
10. Intercellular communication.	25	25	D15(RS3), D16(RS3), D10
11. Gap junctions.	28	24	J19(RS3)
CHAPTER 5: PHYSIOLOGY OF GENETICS AND APOPTOSIS			
Short Answer			
1. What is apoptosis?	37	17	D07(RS2), D19(RS3)
Multiple Choice Questions			
1. Nitrogenous bases present in DNA include all, *except:* a. Adenine b. Guanine c. Cytosine d. **Uracil**	31	14	J21(RS4)

Contd...

PHYSIOLOGY

Contd...

	GKPAL	SEMBU	
CHAPTER 6: TRANSPORT ACROSS THE CELL MEMBRANE			
Short Essays			
1. Compare and contrast active transport with facilitated diffusion.	—	32	D14
2. Transport across the cell membrane.	41	28	J18(RS3), J99
3. Enumerate various transport mechanisms across cell membrane. Explain (primary) active transport with an example.	45,50	28, 32	D07(RS2), J12(RS3)
4. Facilitated diffusion—define and factors affecting it.	47	30	D13(RS3), J16(RS3)
5. Na^+—K^+ pump.	51	33	J08(RS2), J19(RS3)
6. Secondary active transport (define, factors affecting with examples).	53	34	D12(RS3), J14(RS3), J15(RS3)
7. Exocytosis and endocytosis.	54,55	35,36	J13(RS3)
8. Explain endocytosis.	54	35	D08
9. Describe the different steps of phagocytosis.	55	35	D01, D12
Short Answers			
1. What is difference between diffusion and osmosis? Give an example for each.	45,48	—	J02
2. Name 'voltage gated' channels and 'ligand gated' channels.	42	29	J05
3. Explain ligand gated channel with example.	42	29	D03
4. Compare and contrast active transport mechanism and passive transport mechanism.	45	32	D02, J03, J14
5. Simple diffusion.	45	29	D14(RS3)
6. Four factors affecting rate of (simple) diffusion across cell membrane.	45	29	D10, D13
7. Explain facilitated diffusion with an example. How does it differ from simple diffusion.	47	30	J05(RS2), D09(RS2), J11(RS2), J17(RS3), J19(RS3), J04, J10, J13

Contd...

Contd...

	GKPAL	SEMBU	
8. What is active transport? Give examples.	50	32	J00
9. Define 'primary active transport'. Give an example of primary active transport in the cell membrane. What is its function?	51	32	D12, D15
10. What is the function of calcium ATPase pump?	52	33	D05
11. Secondary active transport.	53	34	J06(RS2), J11(RS2), D17(RS3), N20(RS3)
12. Explain exocytosis and endocytosis with an example for each.	54, 55	35, 36	D09(RS2), J17(RS3), D01, D04, D09
13. Explain the mechanism of endocytosis with an example.	54	35	D10(RS2), J10
14. Describe steps of exocytosis.	55	36	J12
15. Phagocytosis (mechanism and stages).	55	35	J07(RS2), D19(RS3), J98, J99, J11

PHYSIOLOGY

CHAPTER 7: MEMBRANE POTENTIAL

Short Essays

1. In a tabular column compare 'local potential' and 'action potential'.	—	708	J05(RS2)
2. Resting membrane potential and genesis (ionic basis).	60	—	D06(RS2), J07(RS2), D10(RS2), D12

Short Answer

1. Resting membrane potential and its ionic basis.	60	—	D09(RS2), J17(RS3), J98, D06, D13

CHAPTER 8: BODY FLUIDS

Short Essays

1. Body fluid compartments.	65,66	47	J09(RS2), D18(RS3)

Contd...

Contd...

	GKPAL	SEMBU	
2. What is extracellular fluid volume (ECF) and how is it measured?	67	47	D08
3. Classify the fluid compartments of body giving their normal values. Mention two methods to determine ECF.	65,66	47	J01
4. Name two principles to determine volume of body fluid compartments.	67	47	J05
5. Briefly describe a method for determination of total body water.	67	47	D05

Short Answers

1. What is the normal plasma osmolarity?	—	—	D06(RS2)
2. Classify body fluid compartments. Give their normal values.	65,66	47	J15(RS3), J04
3. What is the normal ICF volume and ECF volume? Mention any one method for the determination of the same.	67	47	J02
4. What is the normal value of extracellular fluid volume? Name one substance used to measure it.	67	47	J07, J14
5. Name the constituents of ECF and ICF. List four differences between composition of intracellular and extracellular fluid.	68	47	J13(RS3), D03
6. Two methods of determination of ECF.	67	47	D99
7. Explain one method of determination of plasma volume in man.	66	47	D02

SECTION 2: BLOOD AND IMMUNITY

CHAPTER 9: INTRODUCTION TO BLOOD AND PLASMA PROTEINS

Long Essays

1. Enumerate the plasma proteins along with their site of synthesis. List the important functions of plasma proteins and their normal serum levels. Define hypoproteinemia and discuss its clinical significances/add a note on albumin-globulin ratio.	75	55,58	J08(RS2), D09(RS2), D10(RS2), J17(RS3)
2. Explain how plasma albumin determines fluid movement across capillaries. Name four other functions of plasma proteins.	75	56	J04

Contd...

Contd...

	GKPAL	SEMBU	
Short Essays			
1. How much is normal blood volume and how is it kept constant?	—	53	D08
2. Describe one method for determining blood volume.	74	53	D05
3. Plasma proteins—enumerate, functions.	75	56	D14(RS3), D15(RS3), D18(RS3), J19(RS3), J98, D99, D10, D16
Short Answers			
1. What is colloidal osmotic pressure and its significance?	75	56	D11(RS3)
2. What is plasmapheresis? What is its importance?	—	57	J01, J03, D06
3. Give the value of normal blood volume in adults. Explain the principles of measurement of blood volume.	74	53	53, D06(RS2)
4. Functions of plasma proteins.	75	56	J16(RS3), J06, D07, D09
5. Name three important plasma proteins. Give one important function of each.	75	56	D05(RS2)
6. Name the plasma proteins. How much pressure exerted by these proteins in vascular system? What is the importance of this pressure?	75	56	J08
7. Give the normal concentration and function of albumin.	75	56	D98, D13

CHAPTER 10: BONE MARROW AND HEMOPOIESIS

None

CHAPTER 11: RED BLOOD CELLS

Short Essays			
1. Explain the effect of shape of RBC on osmotic fragility. Name two conditions where osmotic fragility is increased.	88	49	D05

Contd...

Contd...

	GKPAL	SEMBU	
2. Packed cell volume (PCV).	88	53	D99
3. Erythrocyte sedimentation rate.	89	76	J12(RS3), J98

Short Answers

1. What is packed cell volume (hematocrit) and how is it determined? Give its significance.	88	53	D11(RS3), J04
2. Erythrocyte sedimentation rate (normal ESR, factors influencing it and its clinical importance).	89	76	J07(RS2), J01, J02, J06, J12

Multiple Choice Questions

1. The sedimentation rate of erythrocyte in not influenced by a. Shape of RBC b. **Volume of RBC** c. Size of Rouleaux d. Globulin content of blood	89	76	J21(RS4)

CHAPTER 12: ERYTHROPOIESIS

Long Essay

1. What is erythropoiesis? Name the sites of erythropoiesis in an adult. Describe the stages/process of erythropoiesis. Briefly describe the factors affecting erythropoiesis. How is this process regulated?	90	64-67	J06(RS2), J14(RS3), D18(RS3), D98, J99, D00, D02, D13

Short Essays

1. Compare the RBC from patients with B_{12} and iron deficiency stages.	—	—	J07
2. Describe the stages of erythropoiesis with their characteristic features. Mention the sites where erythropoiesis occurs.	90	65,66	D99, J07, J14
3. List the changes in erythroid precursors during maturation. Explain the basis of macrocytic anemia.	90	66,67	J04
4. Describe the factors responsible for synthesis and maturation of red blood cells.	94	68,69	D09
5. List six erythropoietic factors. Specify the effects when any two are deficient.	94	68, 69	J05

Contd...

Contd...

	GKPAL	SEMBU	
6. Describe the effect of hypoxia and vitamin B_{12} deficiency on erythropoiesis and erythrocytes.	97,95	67,68	—
7. Explain why vitamin B_{12} deficiency causes anemia. Give the blood picture in this condition.	95	69	D06(RS2)
8. Draw a flowchart to show the regulation of erythropoiesis. List four dietary substances needed for erythropoiesis.	94,95	68,69	J05(RS2)
Short Answers			
1. Enumerate the stages of erythropoiesis. Describe the fate of RBC.	90,101	65,66	D07, D11
2. Describe a polychromatophilic normoblast and gives its significance.	93	66	D03
3. Four factors influencing erythropoiesis.	94	68,69	D99, D14
4. Erythropoietin (sources, action and regulation).	94	68	J07(RS2), J08(RS2), D03
5. Name the maturation factors in erythropoiesis.	94	69	D08
6. What are the effects of vitamin B_{12} and folic acid on erythropoiesis?	95	69	D10
7. Intrinsic factor of castle—secretion and action (physiological significance).	95,96	69	D16(RS3), D08, D13
8. What is reticulocytes? What does reticulocytosis indicate?	93	67	J02
9. Differentiate reticulocyte from erythrocyte.	93	67	D14
Multiple Choice Questions			
1. Erythropoiesis starts in the third week of intrauterine life in: a. Liver b. Spleen c. Bone marrow d. **Mesoderm of the yolk sac**	90	64	J21(RS4)

CHAPTER 13: DESTRUCTION OF RED BLOOD CELLS

Short Essay			
1. Describe the fate of hemoglobin of the damaged red blood corpuscle following hemolysis.	100	72	D15(RS3), J00, J03, J06

Contd...

PHYSIOLOGY

Contd...

	GKPAL	SEMBU	
CHAPTER 14: HEMOGLOBIN AND BLOOD INDICES			
Short Essay			
1. Describe steps in hemoglobin synthesis. Add a note on disorders of hemoglobin synthesis. Mention two types of hemoglobinopathies.	105	71,72	J00
Short Answers			
1. Types of hemoglobin.	105	71	J18(RS3)
2. Fetal hemoglobin.	105	71	J13(RS3)
3. What are the structural and functional differences between adult and fetal hemoglobin?	105	71	D00
4. Mention the functions of hemoglobin.	106	70	D08(RS2), D10(RS2)
5. Define and give the normal values for MCV, MCH and MCHC.	108	79	D00, J15
6. Calculate MCV and MCH, given; PCV= 45%, RBC count = 5 million/cu.mm, Hb%= 15 g%.	108	79	D12(RS3)
7. Explain color index and its significance.	108	79	D10
CHAPTER 15: PATHOPHYSIOLOGY OF ANEMIA AND POLYCYTHEMIA			
Long Essay			
1. What is anemia? Describe different types of anemia with their physiological causes.	110	81,82	J11
Short Essays			
1. Mention the causation, morphological features of red cells and treatment of pernicious anemia.	—	83	J11(RS2)
2. Macrocytic anemia.	111	83	J15(RS3)
3. Classify anemia based on blood indices. Explain any one type of anemia.	110	81	D12
4. Hemolytic anemia.	112	82	N20(RS3)
Short Answers			
1. State the differences between beta thalassemia major and minor.	112	83	D09

Contd...

Contd...

	GKPAL	SEMBU	
2. B_{12} deficiency anemia—give two salient features.	112	83	D14
3. List two features and treatment of macrocytic anemia.	111	83	D16
4. Anemia—define and classify (laboratory/ morphological) an example for each.	110	81	J06(RS2), J12(RS3), J19(RS3)
5. Iron deficiency anemia—important features, blood indices values.	112	83	D13(RS3), D15(RS3)
6. What is meant by aplastic anemia? What is its clinical importance?	112	83	D01, D04
7. Sickle cell anemia.	112	82	D18(RS3), J10

CHAPTER 16: BLOOD GROUPS AND PHYSIOLOGICAL BASIS OF BLOOD TRANSFUSION

Long Essays

1. Explain the basis for classification of blood groups. Describe the Rh blood group system with its importance.	116,120	124,125	J03
2. Classify blood groups and explain how erythroblastosis fetalis takes place.	116,120	124,126	J08
3. Define jaundice. Enumerate the causes of Jaundice. What is hemolytic disease of the newborn? Discuss in brief.	652,120	127, 128, 129	J10(RS2)

Short Essays

1. What is the basis of classification blood groups? Define and explain how Landsteiner's law is applicable to the blood group systems.	116,119	124	D11(RS3)
2. Rhesus factor (Rh factor) and its significance. Add a note on erythroblastosis fetalis.	119	126,129	J06(RS2), D07(RS2), J19(RS3), D14
3. Erythroblastosis foetalis (Rh incompatibility in newborn)—cause, effects (manifestations), treatment (basis and principles) and methods for preventing.	120	126, 129	J21(RS4), D12(RS3), N20(RS3), J98, D98, D03, J10

Contd...

Contd...

	GKPAL	SEMBU	
4. What is meant by mismatched blood transfusion and explain the complications (consequences) of mismatched blood transfusion.	124	127	F21(RS4), D06(RS2), D13(RS3), D17(RS3), N20(RS3), J02, D02, D04, J15
Short Answers			
1. Write briefly the importance of blood groups.	116	125	J08
2. What is Bombay blood group?	118	130	J12(RS3)
3. Name the agglutinogens and agglutinins present in blood in a person of O +ve group. What is "bombay blood group"?	117,118	125, 130	J07(RS2)
4. State Landsteiner's law. Indicate to which blood group system it is not fully applicable.	119	124	D05(RS2), D09(RS2), J18(RS3), D01, D04, J11, J12, J14
5. Give the agglutinogen and agglutinin content of different blood groups of ABO System.	117	125	J13
6. Name the agglutinogens and agglutinins in the following blood types: (a) AB negative; (b) O positive.	117	125	D03
7. Describe erythroblastosis fetalis (hemolytic disease of newborn)—prevention and treatment.	125	129	J01, D02, J11
8. Kernicterus.	121	129	D16(RS3)
9. What is neonatal jaundice? What is the role of phototherapy in its treatment?	120	235	D09
10. Define exchange transfusion. Mention two indications.	121	132	J05
11. Explain why people with 'O' blood group are called universal donors?	123	126	J10
12. Cross matching (define, types).	123	126	D15(RS3)

Contd...

Contd...

	GKPAL	SEMBU	
13. Mismatched blood transfusion—complications (effects).	124	127	D19(RS3), D99, D12
14. What is the mechanism of acute renal failure in mismatched blood transfusion reaction?	124	127	D16

CHAPTER 17: LEUKOPOIESIS

Long Essay

1. Classify leukocytes. Give an account of development (various stages of leukopoiesis) and functions of different leukocytes.	128,137	95	J18(RS3), J13

CHAPTER 18: WHITE BLOOD CELLS

Long Essay

1. Classify the leukocytes and describe their morphological features with the help of diagrams. Elaborate the steps involved in the phagocytic function of neutrophils.	134,137	88,89,90	J11(RS2)

Short Essays

1. T cells versus B cells.	—	—	J08(RS2)
2. Write a short note on functions of leukocytes.	137	91	J14
3. Macrophages—functions.	143	91	D14

Short Answers

1. List the functions of WBCs.	137	91	F21(RS4)
2. Classify lymphocytes based on function and specify their roles.	144	94	J05
3. List the functions of neutrophils.	137	91	D17(RS3)
4. Chemotaxis.	138	93	J15(RS3)
5. What is opsonization and its purpose? Name few opsonins.	138	103	D11(RS3)
6. Eosinophil.	139	89, 93	J15(RS3)
7. Mention the functions of basophils.	141	93	D10
8. Monocytes—morphology and functions.	143	94	D06(RS2), J10
9. How macrophages are derived and what are their function?	143	99	D15

Contd...

Contd...

	GKPAL	SEMBU	
CHAPTER 19: THYMUS AND LYMPHOID TISSUES			
None			
CHAPTER 20: PHYSIOLOGY OF IMMUNITY			
Long Essays			
1. Classify Immunity. Explain the role of B and T lymphocytes in immunity.	156,162	97,98	J21(RS4)
2. Classify T lymphocytes. Explain the mechanism of cellular immunity.	162,165	97,98,99	J16(RS3)
3. Describe in detail the mechanism of antigen recognition and activation of specific immune response in both humoral and cell-mediated immunity. How does HIV disease compromise immunity?	177	106	D15
Short Essays			
1. What is immunity? Describe specific and nonspecific immunity.	156,157	97	D06
2. Define 'innate immunity'. Mention the factors that contribute to the same.	157	97	D13(RS3)
3. What is reticuloendothelial (monocyte—macrophage) system? Outline its function.	158	136	D14(RS3), D17(RS3), J02, J15
4. Macrophage system.	158	99	J13(RS3)
5. T lymphocyte—functions.	162	97,98	J09(RS2), D12(RS3), D16(RS3), D17(RS3), J07, D16
6. Cell-mediated immunity.	165	99	D05(RS2)
7. Explain the role of lymphocytes in immunity.	173	99	J00, J01, J06
8. Humoral immunity—mechanism.	167	101	N20(RS3), D07
9. Explain the role of 'B' lymphocytes in immunity.	163	101	D10
10. Explain the role of complement system in immunity.	169	103	F21(RS4)

Contd...

PHYSIOLOGY

Contd...

	GKPAL	SEMBU	
11. Describe the formation and functions of immunoglobulins.	171	103	D05
Short Answers			
1. What is active and passive immunity? Give one example for each.	—	104	D00
2. What is immunity? Mention the two types of immunity.	156	97	D99
3. Explain the basis of enhanced immune response to booster doses of vaccine.	163	—	F21(RS4)
4. Reticuloendothelial system.	158	136	J08(RS2)
5. List the cells and functions of reticulo/ endothelial system.	158	136	D11
6. Explain acquired immunity.	160	96,98	D07(RS2), J14
7. T lymphocyte—types, functions.	161	97,98	D09(RS2), J17(RS3), D03
8. Give the functions of helper T cell.	162	100	J11
9. List the functions of 'B' lymphocytes.	163	99	D14(RS3), J15
10. Plasma cells.	168	102	D05(RS2), D00, J03, D03
11. What are immunoglobulins? What are their functions.	171	102	D00, D01, D04
12. Draw a diagram showing components of IgG molecule.	171	102	D16

CHAPTER 21: ORGAN TRANSPLANTATION AND APPLIED ASPECTS OF IMMUNITY

Short Answer			
1. Autoimmune phenomenon.	176	106,107	J06(RS2), D06

CHAPTER 22: INTRODUCTION TO HEMOSTASIS, THROMBOPOIESIS AND STRUCTURE, AND PROPERTIES OF PLATELETS

Long Essay			
1. What are platelets? Describe the process of blood coagulation. Name any two anticoagulants and describe their mode of action.	183, 197, 205	109, 113, 118, 119	D06

Contd...

PHYSIOLOGY

Contd...

	GKPAL	SEMBU	
Short Essays			
1. Temporary hemostasis.	181	113	J14(RS3)
2. Platelets.	183	109	J99
3. Describe briefly the functions of thrombocytes.	186	111	D19(RS3), D98, D01
Short Answers			
1. What is megakaryocyte? Where it is present? Briefly write its function.	182	65	D08
2. Describe the morphology of platelets	183	109	J12
3. Functions of platelets (thrombocytes).	186	111	D05(RS2), D09(RS2), D12(RS3), J14(RS3), J17(RS3)
4. What is the normal platelet count? Give two functions of platelets.	186	111	D17(RS3)

CHAPTER 23: ROLE OF PLATELETS IN HEMOSTASIS AND APPLIED ASPECTS OF PLATELETS

Short Essay			
1. Explain the role of platelets in hemostasis.	202	111	D07(RS2)
Short Answers			
1. Explain the mechanism of platelet aggregation.	186	111	J10
2. Name two tests to assess platelet function and give normal value of each.	191	121	J04
3. Purpura.	191	123	D18(RS3)
4. Thrombocytopenic purpura.	191	123	J10(RS2), J13(RS3), J08
5. Purpura and hemophilia.	191, 209	123	D09(RS2)

CHAPTER 24: BLOOD COAGULATION

Long Essays			
1. Define hemostasis. Describe the stages of hemostasis. Describe the mechanism of blood coagulation.	181,197	113, 114, 116, 117	D09

Contd...

Contd...

	GKPAL	SEMBU	
2. Enumerate coagulation factors. Describe the intrinsic and extrinsic mechanism of coagulation with a neat flowchart. Add a note on anticoagulants/Add a note on hemophilia (commonly occurring bleeding disorders)/Add a note on tests for coagulation.	195, 198, 205, 207, 209	116, 117, 118, 119, 121, 123	J07(RS2), D08(RS2), J12(RS3), J15(RS3), D16(RS3), J01, D04, D07
Short Essays			
1. Name the procoagulants and explain how these hasten the coagulation process.	—	121	J09
2. Name the clotting factors and add a note on purpura.	195,191	106, 123	D11
3. Intrinsic mechanism of blood coagulation.	197	117	D10(RS2), D14(RS3), J18(RS3), J12, D13
4. Draw a schematic diagram to show the steps in the intrinsic pathway of blood clotting. Name the mechanisms that initiate this pathway in vivo and in vitro. Add a note on bleeding time.	198	117	D19(RS3), D03
5. Describe the extrinsic pathway of clotting.	198	117	J13
6. Describe the process and significance of clot retraction.	199	111	J07
7. Give a note on fibrinolytic system.	200	118	D10
8. Mechanism of fibrinolysis.	200	118	J16(RS3)
9. Describe the factors maintaining fluidity of blood in the intact vascular system and the factors favoring tendency for clot formation.	201	106, 118, 119	D15
10. Describe the naturally occurring mechanisms which normally prevent clotting.	202	118, 119	J05(RS2)
Short Answers			
1. List two causes of increased bleeding time.	—	123	D14
2. List the natural mechanisms responsible for arrest of bleeding from small blood vessels.	201	116	J05
3. Coagulation factors.	195	116	J10(RS2)

Contd...

Contd...

	GKPAL	SEMBU	
4. Mention the role of factor VII and factor XIII in clotting mechanism. What is hemophilia?	195, 196, 209	123	D12
5. Draw a flowchart showing extrinsic mechanism of clot formation.	198	117	D16
6. Plasmin.	201	118	J98
7. Mention any four factors that prevent coagulation of blood inside the blood vessels.	202	118, 119	J03

CHAPTER 25: ANTICOAGULANTS AND APPLIED ASPECTS OF BLOOD COAGULATION

Short Essays

1. Anticoagulants and their mode of action.	205	118,119	D05(RS2), D09(RS2), D19(RS3), J99, D01, J15
2. What is the normal bleeding time? Name one condition where it is prolonged.	207	121,123	J14
3. A 16-year-old boy was brought to the hospital with excessive bleeding from an injury in his foot. He had a past history of similar delayed stoppage of bleeding associated with swelling of injured parts following blunt trauma. One of his paternal uncles also had a similar history. Investigation revealed: Hb—14 g/dL, platelet count—3.5 lakhs/mm3, BT—5 minutes, CT—12 minutes. a. Mention the probable diagnosis and cause for the same. b. Mention the type of inheritance of this disorder. c. Name another bleeding disorder with the cause.	209	123	F21(RS4)
4. Give a brief account of hemophilia.	209	123	J00, D00, J02, J14

Short Answers

1. Anticoagulants.	205	118,119	J19(RS3), D13

Contd...

Contd...

	GKPAL	SEMBU	
2. Name two anticoagulants with their mechanism of action.	205	118,119	D13(RS3), D14(RS3)
3. Name two anticoagulants used in the laboratory and explain the mechanism of action of any one.	205	119,120	J04
4. Heparin and two actions of heparin as anticoagulant.	206	119	J06
5. Explain how (a) Dicoumarol and (b) EDTA prevent blood clotting.	205	120	D02
6. How does heparin act as an anticoagulant?	206	120	D15
7. What is prothrombin time? Explain its usefulness as a hemostatic test.	208	121	D06(RS2)
8. Name two bleeding disorders. What is von Willebrand's factor?	209,195	123	D07(RS2)
9. Classify hemophilia and its causes of each.	209	123	J08
10. Describe classical hemophilia.	209	123	J99, D07, J10, J15

SECTION 3: NERVE AND MUSCLE

PART A: NERVE

CHAPTER 26: STRUCTURE AND FUNCTIONS OF NEURONS

Short Essay

1. Myelinogenesis.	217	704	J10(RS2)

Short Answers

1. Give a note on myelinogenesis.	217	704	D10
2. Myelination and its physiological significance.	218	704	J05, J15

CHAPTER 27: NERVE POTENTIALS AND PROPAGATION OF NERVE IMPULSE

Short Essays

1. Explain the response of a neuron to the application of a threshold stimulus.	—	160, 708	J12
2. Define chronaxic, rehobase and utilization tissue. Draw a strength duration curve.	227	160	J02, J03, D04

Contd...

PHYSIOLOGY

Contd...

	GKPAL	SEMBU	
3. Explain the strength duration curve.	227	160	D14
4. Action potential in the nerve—describe with a diagram, electrical changes and ionic basis of different phases, properties.	227	708,709	D08(RS2), D17(RS3), D02, J06, D06, D14
5. Draw a sketch of nerve action potential, label its components and explain their causation.	228	708,709	D15
6. Draw and label a nerve action potential. Explain propagation of action potential along an unmyelinated axon.	228, 233	708,710	J13, D16
7. Refractory period.	231	710	J10(RS2)
8. Describe the transmission of impulse in myelinated and non-myelinated nerve fibers (propagation of nerve impulse).	232, 233	704,710	D98, J09, D13
9. Enumerate the sequence of event involved in the transmission of nerve impulse (saltatory conduction).	233	710	F21(RS4), D14(RS3), D98
Short Answers			
1. List four factors that influence conduction in nerve fibers.	—	704	J04
2. What is Quantal summation? Basis of quantal summation.	—	710	D15(RS3), J04
3. What are the characteristics of catelectrotonus?	225	—	J05
4. List the properties of graded potential.	226	708	D16
5. Define the terms chronaxie, rheobase and utilization time.	227	160	D08(RS2), J17(RS3), J00, D00, J07, D07, J09, D15
6. Strength—duration curve.	227	160	J09(RS2), N20(RS3), J08
7. Draw a labeled diagram of monophonic nerve action potential in a neuron.	228	173	D99, D08
8. Explain the mechanism of action of local anesthetics.	230	—	D06(RS2)
9. Explain the role of ionic calcium in nerve excitability.	230	708	J05(RS2)

Contd...

Contd...

	GKPAL	SEMBU	
10. Refractory period—define, cause, ionic basis, types and their role.	231	710	J21(RS4), D03, D11
11. Define refractory period of an excitable tissue. Explain how it differs in cardiac and skeletal muscles, what is its significance.	231	168, 710	J03, J10
12. Absolute refractory period—ionic basis and significance.	231	710	J05(RS2), D12(RS3)
13. Describe saltatory conduction. What is its importance? What are its advantages?	233	710	J09(RS2), J18(RS3), D18(RS3), J98, J01, J02, J03, D14
14. Differentiate between local potential and action potential.	233	708	J03, D15

CHAPTER 28: PROPERTIES AND CLASSIFICATION OF NERVE FIBERS, NERVE INJURY AND OTHER APPLIED ASPECTS

Short Essays

1. Classify nerve fibers based on velocity and diameter (Gasser and Erlanger's classification). Mention the factors influencing conduction of velocity of nerve impulse.	237	707	J00, D01, D03, D09, J14
2. Compound action potential. Give basis of its configuration.	237	708	D05(RS2), J04
3. Changes following nerve injury.	238	711, 712, 713	N20(RS3)
4. Explain Wallerian degeneration and regeneration of nerve fibers.	238	712	J21(RS4), D10(RS2), J11(RS2), D19(RS3)
5. List the factors affecting nerve regeneration.	239	713	F21(RS4)

Short Answers

1. Write the two/three differences between A and C type of nerve fiber.	237	707	J16(RS3), J15
2. Properties (electrical) and functions of nerve fibers.	236	708	J06, J07
3. Why a nerve fiber cannot be fatigued?	237	710	F21(RS4)
4. Classify nerve fibers (Erlanger and Gasser classification).	237	707	J07(RS2), J06

Contd...

Contd...

	GKPAL	SEMBU	
5. Which are the large diameter myelinated nerve fibers according to Erlanger and Gasser's classification? Describe the mode of transmission of impulse in myelinated nerves.	233, 237	707	D11(RS3)
6. Explain what is compound action potential.	237	708	J12
7. Distal changes in the axon following nerve injury (Wallerian degeneration).	238	712	D07(RS2), D15(RS3), D16(RS3), D99
8. What is 'chromatolysis'? When does it occur?	239	712, 713	J13

PART B: NEUROMUSCULAR JUNCTION

CHAPTER 29: NEUROMUSCULAR TRANSMISSION

Long Essay

1. Define myoneural (neuromuscular) junction. Describe the structure of neuromuscular junction and the mechanism of transmission of impulse across neuromuscular junction of skeletal muscle with the help of a diagram. Write about the factors affecting transmission at myoneural junction.	242	181	J10(RS2), J11(RS2), J12(RS3), D16(RS3), J11

Short Essays

1. Neuromuscular junction.	242	181	J18(RS3), J99
2. Explain the mechanism of neuromuscular transmission (sequence of events). Add a note on neuromuscular blockers (name one with mechanism of action).	243	181,182	J05(RS2), J15(RS3), J16(RS3), J19(RS3), D99, J02, J04, D04, D10
3. Neuromuscular blocking agents (classify and explain mechanism of actions).	245	182	D08(RS2), J17(RS3), D18(RS3), J98, J10
4. What is myasthenia gravis? What are its causes and clinical features? Explain the physiological basis of its treatment.	246	192	J06(RS2), D12(RS3), J00, D02, J05, J12

Contd...

Contd...

	GKPAL	SEMBU	
Short Answers			
1. Mention neurotransmitter released and the disease that occurs at neuromuscular junction.	244	181	J06(RS2)
2. Write steps showing fate of acetylcholine at neuromuscular junction.	244	729	J14(RS3)
3. Explain what is end-plate potential.	244	182	J09
4. Neuromuscular blocking agents—classify with one example each, clinical uses.	245	182	D03, D12
5. What is the mechanism of action of botulinum toxin?	245	182	D05
6. Explain the mechanism of action of curare.	245	182	D05(RS2)
7. Name two anticholinesterase drugs acting at neuromuscular junction.	246	182	D15
8. Describe the mechanism of action of a non-depolarizing neuromuscular blocker.	246	—	D05
9. Myasthenia gravis (cause and the physiological basis of cure).	246	192	J98, J99, D01, D04, J08, D13, D14
10. Briefly explain denervation super/hyper-sensitivity.	247	182	D14(RS3), D16(RS3), J05
PART C: MUSCLES			
CHAPTER 30: STRUCTURE OF SKELETAL MUSCLE: PHYSIOLOGICAL ASPECTS			
Short Essays			
1. Draw diagrams to compare the sarcomere at rest and during contraction.	254	156	D05(RS2)
2. Describe the organization and function of sarcotubular system in the skeletal muscle.	254	156	D11(RS3), D14(RS3)
Short Answers			
1. Explain what is 'relaxing proteins' in skeletal muscle.	—	—	J12
2. Compare the role of troponin and calmodulin.	—	—	D06(RS2)

Contd...

PHYSIOLOGY

Contd...

	GKPAL	SEMBU	
3. Muscle proteins and their functions.	251	155	D10(RS2), D00, J07
4. Name the contractile proteins present in the muscle.	251	155	J10
5. Troponin.	253	157	J99
6. Sarcomere (draw in relaxed and contracted state).	253	155	J06(RS2), J11(RS2), J15(RS3), D19(RS3), J98, D00, J01, D01, J04, D04, J08, D11
7. Mention the components and functions of sarcotubular system in skeletal muscle (draw a labeled diagram).	255	157,158	J01, J13, D16
8. Write about storage, release, functions and reuptake of ionic calcium in skeletal muscle.	256	—	J16(RS3)

CHAPTER 31: EXCITATION-CONTRACTION COUPLING AND MOLECULAR BASIS OF SKELETAL MUSCLE CONTRACTION

Long Essays

1. Describe the structure of a skeletal muscle. Explain the molecular basis of skeletal muscle contraction.	254, 258	156,175	D10
2. What is a sarcomere? Describe the molecular basis of muscular contraction (excitation contraction coupling) in skeletal muscle. Add a note on myasthenia gravis.	246, 254, 258	155, 175, 192	J06
3. Describe the molecular basis of skeletal muscle contraction. Add a note on isometric contraction.	258,263	161,175	J14(RS3)
4. Describe the excitation—contraction coupling in skeletal muscle. What is the phenomenon of muscle fatigue?	258,269	175	J07(RS2)
5. Describe the molecular basis of muscular contraction in skeletal muscle. Add a note on features seen in fatigue of a muscle.	258,269	175	N20(RS3), J15

Short Essays

1. Electromyogram.	—	190	D10(RS2)

Contd...

Contd...

	GKPAL	SEMBU	
2. Describe the sarcotubular system. Explain the excitation contraction coupling the skeletal muscle.	254, 258	157, 175	D06
3. Explain the (sliding filament) mechanism of muscle contraction.	258	175	D15(RS3), J13
4. Explain excitation-contraction coupling reaction with help of a diagram.	258	175	D09(RS2), J18(RS3), J99, D01, J03, D11
5. Role of calcium in muscle contraction.	259	175	D08(RS2), J15(RS3)
6. Walk along mechanism for contraction of muscle (molecular basis of muscle contraction).	258	175	D07(RS2), J08(RS2), J01, J10, D16
7. Explain the ratchet theory of muscle contraction.	258	175	J21(RS4)
8. Isotonic and isometric contraction in skeletal muscle—define, describe the differences giving examples for each.	263	161	J17(RS3), D05, D12
9. Explain two different ways by which force of contraction of skeletal muscle is increased in the body.	263	162	D03
Short Answers			
1. Explain electromyography and its clinical importance.	—	190	J09
2. Electromyogram (EMG).	—	190	D12(RS3), D17(RS3)
3. What are fibrillations and fasciculations? How are these recorded?	—	190,192	D07
4. What is isometric and isotonic contraction? Differentiate isometric and isotonic muscle contraction with one example for each.	263	161	D00, J02, J03, D08, D11, D14

CHAPTER 32: SKELETAL MUSCLE: PROPERTIES, FIBER TYPES, AND APPLIED ASPECTS

Short Essays			
1. Explain the refractory periods in skeletal muscle.	—	168	D07

Contd...

PHYSIOLOGY

Contd...

	GKPAL	SEMBU	
2. Explain temporal and spatial summation in muscle.	—	—	J05(RS2)
3. Enumerate the properties of skeletal muscle. Explain the property of fatigue in detail and factors affecting it.	265,269	265,269	D11
4. Explain the length tension relationship in skeletal muscle.	267	167	D06(RS2)
5. Fatigue—define, sites, causes and effects of muscle fatigue, factors affecting. What is contraction remainder or physiological contracture? Why does the cardiac muscle not become fatigued?	269	163	D11(RS3), J08
6. Differentiate between red and white muscles.	270	160, 162	D11
7. What is motor unit and how it is formed?	270	183	J11
Short Answers			
1. Refractory period in skeletal muscle.	—	168	D18(RS3)
2. What are the functions of ATP in skeletal muscle contraction?	268	177	D09, J14
3. Compare and contrast red (slow/type I) and white (fast/type II) muscle fibers.	270	162	F21(RS4), J21(RS4), D16
4. Explain the causes of heat rigor and rigor mortis.	269	165	D09, J14
5. Rigor mortis—define, mechanism, medicolegal importance.	269	165	J19(RS3), D98, J01, D02, D03, J10, J12
6. Motor unit—define, significance (of such arrangement in skeletal muscle), recruitment.	270	183	J05(RS2), D11(RS3), D14(RS3), J17(RS3), D19(RS3), D98, D00, J07, D14, J15
7. Explain how asynchronous discharge of motor units is helpful.	271	—	D16

Contd...

Contd...

	GKPAL	SEMBU	
CHAPTER 33: SMOOTH MUSCLE AND CARDIAC MUSCLE			
Short Essays			
1. Describe the differences between the two types of smooth muscle.	274	186	J05
2. Describe the mechanism of smooth muscle contraction (excitation-contraction coupling in visceral smooth muscle).	277	188	D08, J09
3. Name the properties of smooth muscle. How do you explain the semi-rhythmicity in smooth muscle?	278	186	D07
4. Functional properties of smooth muscle.	278	186	D15(RS3)
5. In a tabular form, give the differences between skeletal, cardiac and smooth muscle.	280	152	D05
6. Compare and contrast skeletal muscle with cardiac muscle (two functional differences).	280	152	J16(RS3), D13
7. Five differences between smooth muscle and cardiac muscle.	280	152	J06(RS2), J15(RS3)
Short Answers			
1. Functions of smooth muscle.	—	184	D18(RS3)
2. Name the two major types of smooth muscles. Give any two differences between them.	274	186	J13
3. Enumerate the properties of (visceral) smooth muscle.	278	186	D05(RS2), D99, D08
4. Differences between skeletal muscle and smooth muscle.	280	152	D17(RS3)
SECTION 4: AUTONOMIC NERVOUS SYSTEM			
CHAPTER 34: FUNCTIONAL ORGANIZATION OF AUTONOMIC NERVOUS SYSTEM			
Short Essay			
1. Cholinergic sympathetic fibers.	285	885	D10(RS2)
CHAPTER 35: SYMPATHETIC SYSTEM			
Short Essay			
1. Enumerate effects of sympathetic stimulation.	296	885	J14(RS3)

Contd...

Contd...

	GKPAL	SEMBU	
Short Answer			
1. Compare the effects of sympathetic and parasympathetic stimulation on pupil.	296	885	J15

CHAPTER 36: PARASYMPATHETIC SYSTEM

Short Essay

1. Describe the effects of parasympathetic stimulation on cardiac and smooth muscles.	301	885	J10

CHAPTER 37: CONTROL OF AUTONOMIC FUNCTIONS AND APPLIED ASPECTS

None

CHAPTER 38: AUTONOMIC FUNCTION TESTS

None

CHAPTER 39: HEART RATE VARIABILITY

None

CHAPTER 40: BLOOD PRESSURE VARIABILITY AND BAROREFLEX SENSITIVITY

None

SECTION 5: CARDIOVASCULAR SYSTEM

PART A: GENERAL INTRODUCTION

CHAPTER 41: FUNCTIONAL ORGANIZATION OF CARDIOVASCULAR SYSTEM

Long Essay

1. Describe the role of the different types of blood vessels. Explain how it is related to their structure.	332	485	J04

Short Essay

1. Name the different types of blood vessels and give an example for each. Explain the role of any one type.	333	485	J05

Contd...

PHYSIOLOGY

Contd...

	GKPAL	SEMBU	
Short Answers			
1. Types of blood vessels and their significance	332	485	D14
2. What is Windkessel effect? What is its importance/functions?	332	556	J12(RS3), J14(RS3), D16(RS3), D00, D07
3. What are: (a) Resistance vessels, (b) Capacitance vessels, (c) Exchange vessels?	332	485	J01
4. Which segments of vascular system contribute the resistance to blood flow and why? Give the formula relating resistance to pressure and flow.	332, 418	555	D11(RS3)
5. Capacitance vessels.	333	486	J08(RS2)
6. Differences between pulmonary and systemic circulation.	334	487	D05(RS2), D15(RS3)

PART B: HEART

CHAPTER 42: FUNCTIONAL ANATOMY OF HEART, CARDIAC INNERVATION AND CARDIAC MUSCLE

Short Essays			
1. Innervations of the heart.	340	548	D08(RS2)
2. Discuss the length-tension relationship in cardiac muscle.	342	—	D10(RS2)
3. Define Frank Sterling's law of the heart and explain its importance with the help of a graph.	343	535	D12(RS3), D19(RS3)
Short Answers			
1. Explain what is vagal tone? What determines it? Mention its importance.	341	549	J07(RS2), J09(RS2), N20(RS3), J99, D06, D12, D16
2. What are the effects of parasympathetic (vagal) stimulation on heart?	341	549	J11(RS2), D13(RS3)
3. Intercalated disc and its significance.	342	483	D14(RS3), J15
4. Define Sterling's law of muscle contraction. Explain its molecular basis. How it is applied in case of cardiac muscle.	343	535	D00, J01, D02

Contd...

PHYSIOLOGY

Contd...

	GKPAL	SEMBU	
5. Define Frank-Starling's law of heart.	343	535	D05(RS2), D17(RS3), J05

CHAPTER 43: PROPERTIES OF CARDIAC MUSCLE

Long Essay

1. Describe the properties of cardiac muscle.	346	488	D16(RS3), D15

Short Essay

1. Properties of cardiac muscle (enumerate). Explain refractory period in heart muscles (importance of long refractory period).	346	488	J18(RS3), D18(RS3), D19(RS3) D99, D07, J14

Short Answers

1. Mention properties of cardiac muscle.	346	488	J12(RS3)
2. Name the properties of cardiac muscle and what is the importance of absolute refractory period.	346	488	J09
3. Autorhythmicity—physiological basis.	346	489	D17(RS3), D19(RS3)
4. SA node as pacemaker.	347	490	D06
5. Refractory period of a cardiac muscle fiber and its significance.	347	493	J09(RS2), D18(RS3), J15
6. Why the cardiac muscles will not undergo tetanus or fatigue?	348	494	J03
7. Explain "all or none law" with respect to cardiac muscle and skeletal muscles.	349	493	D16(RS3), D19(RS3), D01, D02, D04, D09, J10, J14
8. Define (i) All or none law and (ii) Starling's law.	343, 349	493	D99
9. Define 'all or none law' and 'absolute refractory period'.	344, 349	493	D12
10. What is the mechanism of staircase phenomenon?	349	493	D05

Contd...

Contd...

	GKPAL	SEMBU	
CHAPTER 44: ELECTROPHYSIOLOGY OF THE HEART			
Short Essays			
1. Cardiac action potential (ventricular muscle action potential).	355	488	D10(RS2)
2. Draw and describe cardiac pacemaker potential and explain the ionic basis.	356	491	J12(RS3), D13(RS3), J14(RS3), J07
3. Describe the generation of impulse in sinuatrial node.	356	491	J11
4. Draw a labeled diagram to show the membrane potential of cardiac pacemaker tissue. Explain the effect of vagal stimulation on this potential.	356	491	J04
Short Answers			
1. Draw and label the ventricular muscle action potential	355	488	D02
2. Pacemaker potential (draw and label).	356	491	J13(RS3), D11
3. What is the effect of sympathetic stimulation on pacemaker potential?	357	491	J16(RS3)
CHAPTER 45: CONDUCTING SYSTEM OF HEART; ORIGIN AND SPREAD OF CARDIAC IMPULSE			
Long Essay			
1. Draw a labeled diagram of the conducting system of heart. Describe the conducting system of heart and it importance. Explain the pathway of spread of cardiac impulse. What is AV nodal delay? What is its importance?	359	492	D09(RS2), J17(RS3), J02, D02
Short Essays			
1. Describe with illustration the conducting system of heart and mention velocity of conduction. Mention the significance of AV nodal delay.	359	492	J21(RS4), J15(RS3), J16(RS3), D16(RS3)
2. Draw a diagram and explain the location and role of each part of the conducting system of the human heart.	359	492	J05(RS2), J07(RS2)
3. Draw a diagram of special conducting system of heart. How is idioventricular rhythm produced?	359	492	J09

Contd...

Contd...

	GKPAL	SEMBU	
4. Name the internodal tracts in the conducting system of heart. Explain the importance of AV nodal delay	359,361	492	D08
5. Compare the velocity of conduction in various parts of conducting system of heart. Give the significance of the slowest and fastest parts.	360	492	D03
6. Generation and conduction (mode of propagation) of cardiac impulse over the heart.	360	492	D05(RS2), J01, J03, D10, D14, D15

Short Answers

1. Draw and label the pathway of impulse conduction in heart.	359	492	J11
2. Name the special conducting (junctional) tissues of the heart.	359	492	D99
3. Significance of AV nodal delay.	361	492	J05

CHAPTER 46: ELECTROCARDIOGRAM

Long Essays

1. What is ECG? What is Einthoven's triangle? Enumerate the various ECG leads with a suitable diagram. Describe (draw and label) a normal typical ECG from Lead II. Discuss the various waves, intervals and segments in a normal ECG and their causation (basis) and importance. Add a note on his bundle electrocardiogram. State Einthoven's law.	363, 364, 365, 376	512	J21(RS4), J08(RS2), J11(RS2), D17(RS3), D18(RS3), D06, J07, J09
2. Explain the principle, method of recording, waves and intervals of electrocardiogram. Discuss how an ECG recording helps to evaluate conduction disorders of the heart.	364,376	512	J13(RS3), J06

Short Essays

1. Explain Einthoven's law.	—	521	D13
2. Cardiac arrest.	—	612	J10(RS2)
3. Standard limb leads.	364	513	D08(RS2)
4. Diagrammatically represent a normal ECG. Explain normal waves and causes for different waves.	366	514	D00, J03, D05

Contd...

Contd...

	GKPAL	SEMBU	
5. RR and QT interval in ECG.	366	517	D16
6. QRS complex.	366	516	D15(RS3)
7. PR interval.	366	517	J08(RS2), J09(RS2), D19(RS3),
8. RR interval and its significance.	374	518	D18(RS3)
9. Mean electrical axis of QRS vector.	373	516	D14
10. Paroxysmal tachycardia.	375	528	J10(RS2)
11. Ventricular fibrillation.	375	529	J10(RS2)
12. Heart block.	376	525	J10(RS2)
13. Explain what is incomplete and complete heart block.	376	525	J10
14. Stokes-Adam syndrome.	377	527	J10(RS2)
Short Answers			
1. Einthoven's triangle.	364	520	J06(RS2)
2. What is the role of augmented limb leads?	365	513	D16(RS3)
3. Waves of ECG.	365	514	D07(RS2)
4. List chest leads of ECG. Give their location.	365	514	J12
5. Draw a labeled diagram of normal electrocardiogram recorded from lead II.	366	515	D07(RS2), D10(RS2), D98, D99, J01, D01, D04, J13
6. PR interval in ECG—define, normal value, events occurring, significance.	366	517	D16(RS3), J17(RS3), J19(RS3), J98, J99, D02, D03, D09, D12
7. Importance of QT interval of ECG.	366	517	D13
8. Give the cause of the 'P' wave of the ECG. Explain the abnormalities of `P' wave of ECG. State two conditions which alter this wave.	369	515	J05(RS2), D16
9. What is the cause of 'T' wave in the ECG? In which leads is it inverted normally?	369	517	J09

Contd...

Contd...

	GKPAL	SEMBU	
10. Sinus arrhythmia—define and causes.	372	523	D11(RS3), D12(RS3), D17(RS3)
11. What is bundle of Kent and what ECG changes are demonstrated in its presence?	377	528	D08
12. Mention the symptoms and ECG changes in ischemic heart disease.	377	—	F21(RS4)

CHAPTER 47: CARDIAC CYCLE

Long Essays

1. Define cardiac cycle. Explain with the help of a diagram the mechanical changes during cardiac cycle.	384	495	D15(RS3), J00, J14
2. Explain the phases of a normal cardiac cycle. With the help of a labeled diagram (left ventricular pressure tracing) describe the changes in left ventricular pressure during cardiac cycle.	384	495	D05, D12
3. Mention the events of a cardiac cycle with their duration. Explain the left ventricular pressure and volume changes during cardiac cycle.	384,387	495	F21(RS4)
4. Draw a neat labeled diagram of the cardiac cycle, correlating it with pressure and volume changes. Explain the events in detail.	385	495	J09(RS2)

Short Essays

1. Left ventricular pressure changes.	—	—	D08
2. Describe phonocardiogram.	—	—	J12
3. Give the normal value of end diastolic ventricular volume. Name two factors that increase this volume and explain its significance in ventricular function.	—	502	J05
4. Normal cardiac cycle.	384	495	J99
5. Ventricular events of cardiac cycle.	385	495	D11(RS3), D06
6. Draw the diagram of left ventricular pressure—volume loop and explain the causation of component segments.	385	503	D15

Contd...

Contd...

	GKPAL	SEMBU	
7. Describe right atrial pressure changes during cardiac cycle.	385	498	D10
8. Jugular venous pulse tracing (causes of each wave).	389	500	D09(RS2), J13(RS3), J16(RS3), J17(RS3), J08
9. First and second heart sounds.	390	496,498	J06(RS2)
10. Heart sounds and murmurs.	390	496	J13(RS3), J18(RS3), N20(RS3)
11. How are heart sounds produced? Mention their characteristics and clinical significance?	390	496	D98
12. Tabulate the differences between first and second heart sounds. Add a note on splitting of second heart sound.	390	496,498	D07(RS2)
13. Explain the causes of four heart sounds during cardiac cycle. How are these recorded?	390	496	J08
Short Answers			
1. Write briefly the right ventricular pressure changes during cardiac cycle.	—	501	J09
2. Write briefly on volume changes in the ventricles during cardiac cycle.	—	496	J09
3. Phonocardiogram.	—	—	D12(RS3)
4. Differentiate first and Second heart sounds.	—	496,498	J12(RS3), D14(RS3), J00, J01
5. Jugular venous pulse (labeled diagram).	389	500	J18(RS3), D05
6. Heart sounds (causes).	390	496	J19(RS3), D07
7. First heart sound—describe.	390	496	D11
8. Second heart sound—describe, cause.	390	498	J06, J12
Multiple Choice Questions			
1. Normal duration of protodiastole of cardiac cycle is: a. 0.02 sec b. **0.04 sec** c. 0.08 sec d. 0.12 sec	—	498	J21(RS4)

Contd...

PHYSIOLOGY

Contd...

	GKPAL	SEMBU	
2. Following are the events in ventricular diastole, *except:* a. Isovolumetric relaxation phase b. First rapid filling phase c. Diastasis d. Rapid ejection phase	387	498	J21(RS4)

CHAPTER 48: CARDIAC OUTPUT

Long Essays

1. Define cardiac output. Discuss factors affecting it. Add a note on left ventricular failure.	394,399	532,612	D16
2. Define cardiac output and cardiac index. Give their normal values. Describe the factors, which regulate cardiac output (regulation of cardiac output) and mention various method of its determination. Write a note on cardiac reserve.	394, 404, 396, 395	532, 533, 534	D06(RS2), D13(RS3), J15(RS3), J19(RS3), N20(RS3), J12, J15

Short Essays

1. Define cardiac output and mention the factors regulating it. Describe one method of its measurement.	394, 404, 396	532, 534, 535	J98, D99, J01, D01, J06, J08
2. Define Fick's principle. Give details of estimation of cardiac output based on it.	396	536	J11(RS2)
3. Describe the measurement of cardiac output by dye-dilution technique.	397	538	J10
4. Explain how preload affects cardiac output.	399	534	D12
5. Venous return.	400	534	D12(RS3)
6. Explain factors influencing (promoting) venous returns.	400	534	D11(RS3), D17(RS3), D01

Short Answers

1. Define stroke volume. Give its normal value.	394	532	J14
2. Cardiac index.	394	532	J06(RS2)
3. Ejection fraction.	395	533	N20(RS3)
4. Define cardiac reserve.	395	533	D11
5. Name the methods of measurement of cardiac output.	396	534	D15(RS3)

Contd...

PHYSIOLOGY

Contd...

	GKPAL	SEMBU	
6. State Fick's principle. Explain how it is applied to determine cardiac output.	396	536	J18(RS3), J00, D00, D02, D03, D11
7. Venous return.	400	534	J13(RS3)
8. Name the factors increasing the venous return to right atrium.	400	534	D98, J09

CHAPTER 49: HEART RATE AND ARTERIAL PULSE

Long Essay

1. Describe the baroreceptors control of heart rate. Name six other affecting the heart rate.	408	551, 547	D03

Short Essays

1. What is normal heart rate? How is it regulated (nervous regulation)?	408,409	548	J99, J08
2. Explain the effects of vagal stimulation on heart.	409	549	J13
3. Radial pulse tracing—illustrate and physiological basis.	410	—	F21(RS4)
4. Describe the normal 'arterial pulse' and 'jugular venous pulse'.	410, 389	582	D12
5. Water-hammer pulse.	411	—	D08(RS2)

Short Answers

1. What is bainbridge reflex? What is it's importance?	409	552	D11(RS3), J16(RS3), J01, J02, D02, J11
2. Draw a labeled diagram of arterial pulse.	410	—	J07
3. What is bradycardia? In which subjects is it observed physiologically and explain the reason?	410	547	D08

PART C: CIRCULATION

CHAPTER 50: PRINCIPLES OF HEMODYNAMICS

Short Essays

1. What is Hagen's Poiseuille's law? Write the formula and explain its application.	416	556	J08(RS2), D10(RS2), D14(RS3)

Contd...

Contd...

	GKPAL	SEMBU	
2. Poiseuille-Hagen formula. Name two factors normally alter in it and explain the effect of each.	416	556	J04, D09
3. What is turbulent flow of blood? Where is it taking place physiologically? How it is measured?	416	554	D08
4. Peripheral resistance.	417	555	D99
Short Answers			
1. Write the Poiseuille-Hagen formula and state its importance.	416	556	J05(RS2), J06
2. What is Reynold's number and what is its significance?	416	554	D10(RS2), D10, J15
3. Peripheral resistance and factors influencing it.	417	555	J18(RS3), J99

CHAPTER 51: ARTERIAL SYSTEM

Short Essay

1. Korotkoff's sounds.	423	567	J06(RS2)

CHAPTER 52: CAPILLARY CIRCULATION

Short Essays

1. Capillary circulation.	425	594	D05(RS2)
2. What is microcirculation and explain the pressures in it.	425	594	J09
3. Explain dynamics of capillary fluid exchange. How is it affected in hypoproteinemia.	428	—	D06(RS2)
4. Describe tissue fluid formation and explain two mechanisms which produce edema.	428	144	J05(RS2)
5. Describe Starlings forces affecting fluid exchange in at capillary level. Explain the role of each force acting across capillaries in tissue fluid formation.	428	144	J07
6. Define edema. Describe mechanism of edema.	429	145	D07
Short Answers			
1. Physiological shunt.	—	596	J99

Contd...

Contd...

	GKPAL	SEMBU	
2. List two factors affecting capillary fluid shift.	—	596	J15
3. Name two locations of fenestrated capillaries. Specify their function.	426	—	D03
4. Enumerate four factors affecting tissue fluid formation.	428	—	D14

CHAPTER 53: LYMPHATIC SYSTEM AND LYMPHATIC CIRCULATION

Short Essay

1. What is lymph? Describe the formation and circulation of lymph. What are its functions?	431,432	142	D11(RS3), J18(RS3), J10

Short Answers

1. Explain why edema occurs with blockage of lymph vessels.	429	146	D03
2. Factors affecting flow of lymph.	—	142	D06
3. Functions of lymph.	433	142	D11
4. List the functions of lymphatic circulation.	433	142	J14(RS3)

CHAPTER 54: VENOUS SYSTEM

None.

CHAPTER 55: REGULATION OF BLOOD PRESSURE

Long Essays

1. Define and give normal values of arterial blood pressure, systolic and diastolic blood pressure, mean arterial pressure and pulse pressure. How is it measured? Discuss the (short-term/long-term) factors regulating the blood pressure.	438,439	559, 566, 560	D05(RS2), D07(RS2), D10(RS2), D14(RS3), J98, D08, D14
2. Define systolic and diastolic blood pressure and give their normal values. Explain the baroreceptor reflex mechanism for regulation of blood pressure.	438, 444	559,562	J14(RS3)
3. Describe the role of carotid sinus in the regulation of arterial blood pressure.	444	563,569	D98

Contd...

Contd...

	GKPAL	SEMBU	
Short Essays			
1. Define 'mean arterial pressure' and explain the importance of maintaining it.	439	559,560	D13(RS3)
2. Describe the nervous regulation of blood pressure.	441	561	J12
3. Describe the role of vasomotor center in regulation of arterial blood pressure.	442	562	D10
4. Describe the sinoaortic reflex and its importance.	444	563	J12(RS3), D15(RS3), N20(RS3), D02, J03, D04, D06
5. Baroreceptors.	444	562	J08(RS2)
6. Baroreceptor reflexes.	444	562	J06(RS2)
7. Describe the role of baroreceptors in regulation of blood pressure.	444	562	D13
8. Describe the role of chemoreceptors in regulation of blood pressure.	446	563	J13
9. Describe how Cushing's reflex is activated and its effect on systemic blood pressure.	447	—	J11(RS2)
10. Describe the actions of angiotensin II (in regulation of blood pressure).	450	564	D05, D16
11. Describe the role of different hormones in regulation of blood pressure.	450	564	D09
12. Explain the role of rennin-angiotensin-aldosterone system in BP regulation.	450	564	F21(RS4), J06(RS2), D08(RS2), D00
13. Rennin-angiotensin-aldosterone axis.	450	564	D07(RS2)
14. Long-term regulation of arterial blood pressure.	451	564	J99, J14
Short Answers			
1. Explain the direct effect of CO_2 and hypoxia on vasomotor center.	—	—	D10
2. Find out mean arterial blood pressure, if systolic pressure is 120 mm Hg and diastolic pressure is 90 mm Hg.	—	559	D10
3. Four factors influencing systolic blood pressure.	439	560	D99

Contd...

Contd...

	GKPAL	SEMBU	
4. Name the arterial baroreceptors. How are they stimulated? Mention two effects of stimulation of baroreceptors.	444	562	D06(RS2)
5. Name the baroreceptors regulating blood pressure.	444	562	J15
6. Define Marey's law. What is its basis? Mention one condition which is an exception to this.	446	—	D13(RS3), D00, J03
7. Location and innervation of peripheral chemoreceptors.	446	—	J05
8. What is Cushing's reaction? What is its importance? How it restores blood pressure?	447	—	D01, D04, J08, D14
9. What is importance of renin-angiotensin mechanism?	450	564	J08

CHAPTER 56: INTEGRATED REGULATION OF CARDIOVASCULAR FUNCTIONS

Short Answer

1. Sympathetic and parasympathetic tone.	457	—	J08(RS2)

CHAPTER 57: AN OVERVIEW OF REGIONAL CIRCULATION

Short Essay

1. List the theories of autoregulation of blood flow and explain any two.	461	558	F21(RS4)
2. Draw a labeled graph to show autoregulation of blood flow. Explain any one mechanism by which it occurs.	461	558	J05

Short Answer

1. Define autoregulation of blood flow. Mention three theories which explain it.	461	558	J00, J03

CHAPTER 58: CEREBRAL CIRCULATION

Short Essays

1. Peculiarities of cerebral circulation.	463	589	J17(RS3)
2. Regulation of cerebral circulation (blood flow).	465	590	J07(RS2), J16(RS3), D16(RS3)
3. Describe the mechanism of auto regulation of cerebral blood flow.	465	590	D09

Contd...

PHYSIOLOGY

Contd...

	GKPAL	SEMBU	
Short Answers			
1. Name two techniques to monitor regional blood flow in the brain.	465	589	D03
2. List the factors influencing cerebral circulation.	465	590	J00, D05

CHAPTER 59: CORONARY CIRCULATION

Long Essay			
1. Describe in detail the coronary circulation and the factors influencing it.	469	583,585	D11
Short Essays			
1. Coronary circulation and its special features.	469	583,584	J05(RS2), , D08(RS2), J15(RS3), J98, D98, D06
2. Give the value of resting coronary blood flow and describe the phasic variation of coronary blood flow during cardiac cycle.	469	584,585	D11(RS3)
3. Explain the factors influencing coronary circulation (regulation of coronary circulation).	469	585	D00, D01, J03, J12
4. Describe the mechanism of autoregulation of coronary blood flow.	470	585	D13
5. Role of adenosine in blood flow regulation.	470	586	D08(RS2)
Short Answers			
1. Enumerate the factors governing oxygen consumption by the heart.	—	—	D07(RS2)
2. Explain the phasic nature of coronary blood flow.	469	585	D02, D12
3. List four factors influencing coronary blood flow.	469	585	J14
4. What is 'angina pectoris'? Explain the basis of it with a diagram.	470	587	J07(RS2), J99

Contd...

Contd...

	GKPAL	SEMBU	
CHAPTER 60: CUTANEOUS, SPLANCHNIC AND SKELETAL MUSCLE CIRCULATION			
Short Essays			
1. Describe the characteristic features of cutaneous circulation.	473	598	D13
2. Triple response (reaction).	474	599	J08(RS2), D16(RS3), D11
3. Describe the characteristic features of splanchnic circulation.	475	592	J13
Short Answers			
1. Cutaneous blood flow.	473	598	J07
2. Mention the features of axon reflex with its basis.	474	599	J21(RS4), D15(RS3), J10, J15, D16
3. Triple response.	474	599	J06(RS2), D06(RS2), J09(RS2), D14(RS3), N20(RS3), J98, J99, J00, D00, J02
4. Write a note on skeletal muscle blood flow.	477	597	D11
CHAPTER 61: FETAL AND NEONATAL CIRCULATION			
None			
PART D: APPLIED AND CLINICAL ASPECTS OF CARDIOVASCULAR SYSTEM			
CHAPTER 62: PATHOPHYSIOLOGY OF HYPERTENSION AND HYPOTENSION			
Short Essay			
1. What is meant by Goldblatt hypertension? Explain the underlying mechanism of hypertension.	484	569	D15

Contd...

Contd...

	GKPAL	SEMBU	
Short Answers			
1. What is hypertension? What are the causes leading to secondary hypertension?	483,484	568	J09
2. Physiological basis of a drug in hypertension.	486	570	D10(RS2)
3. What is postural hypotension?	486	570	J16(RS3), D16(RS3)

CHAPTER 63: PATHOPHYSIOLOGY OF SHOCK

Long Essays			
1. Explain the role of arterial baroreceptors soon after blood loss. Name the other compensatory mechanisms available.	—	607	J05(RS2)
2. What is shock? Classify shock. Discuss the various types and physiological basis of treatment.	488,491	606,607	J10(RS2)
3. Describe the circulatory changes to moderate blood loss.	489	607	D13
4. Describe the physiological basis of 'irreversible shock'	490	607	J13
5. Explain the cardiovascular adjustments following: (a) Moderate exercise; (b) Hemorrhage. Add a note on 'irreversible shock'.	489,490	607	J07(RS2)
Short Essays			
1. Define shock. What are the causes of shock? What is meant by irreversible shock?	488,490	606,607	J02, J12
2. List four features of hemorrhagic shock. Explain the basis of any two features.	488	607	J05
Short Answers			
1. Classify types of shock.	488	607	D11
2. Mention four compensatory mechanisms in hypovolemic (circulatory) shock.	489	607	D99
3. Explain the mechanism of refractory shock.	491	607	D09
4. Explain what is irreversible shock?	490	607	D10

Contd...

Contd...

	GKPAL	SEMBU	
CHAPTER 64: PATHOPHYSIOLOGY OF HEART FAILURE			
Short Essay			
1. Describe the manifestations of congestive heart failure.	494	612	J10
Short Answer			
1. Explain the principles of cardiac resuscitation.	—	—	D13
SECTION 6: RESPIRATORY SYSTEM			
CHAPTER 65: FUNCTIONAL ORGANIZATION OF RESPIRATORY SYSTEM			
Short Essays			
1. Explain nonrespiratory functions of lungs.	506	625	D07
2. Functions of upper respiratory passage.	501	—	J07(RS2), D13(RS3)
Short Answers			
1. List the functions of nasal cavity.	502	—	J01, D01, D04
2. Functions of conducting zone of respiratory tree.	503	—	D14
3. List four nonrespiratory functions of respiratory system.	506	625	J06(RS2), D03
CHAPTER 66: MECHANICS OF BREATHING			
Long Essays			
1. With the help of graphs, explain the mechanism of air entry and exit from the lungs.	511	634	J05(RS2)
2. Describe how expansion of thorax is brought about during eupnea.	511	632	D05, D14
3. Describe the mechanics of respiration. Define lung compliance. Mention two conditions which reduce lung compliance.	511,516	632,635	J03, J14
4. Draw a labeled graph to show the lung volumes and capacities and give the normal values of each. Give the significance of volume of air left in lungs after maximal expiration.	513	638,641	D03

Contd...

Contd...

	GKPAL	SEMBU	
Short Essays			
1. Explain why the alveoli remain dry.	—	—	D06
2. Name the muscles of inspiration and expiration. Explain the role of inspiratory and expiratory muscles in normal respiration.	509	631	D15(RS3), J04
3. Give the nerve supply and functional importance of diaphragm.	509	632	D13(RS3)
4. What is the intrapleural pressure? What are the variations in different phases of respiration?	510	634	J09
5. Draw a graph to show changes in intrapleural pressure during a normal respiratory cycle. Explain the basis of the changes.	510	634	J05
6. Describe the mechanics of breathing? What are the factors necessary in automatic breathing?	—	632	J09, J11, J12
7. Draw a labeled diagram showing subdivisions of lung volume.	514	641	D05
8. Draw and explain a spirogram.	514	641	J13(RS3), D19(RS3)
9. Draw a spirogram indicating various lung volumes and capacities.	514	641	J01, J09
10. Vital capacity.	514	639	D14(RS3)
11. Functional residual capacity—define, normal value and measurements.	515	639	F21(RS4)
12. Lung compliance—describe, name factors affecting it, condition where it is increased and decreased.	516	635	D17(RS3), D00, D06, J15
13. Pulmonary surfactant—chemical composition and functions.	520	633	J21(RS4), J14(RS3), J15(RS3), D18(RS3), J19(RS3)
14. Name the source and chemical nature of lung surfactant. Explain its role in respiration. Indicate the consequences when it is deficient.	520	633	J06(RS2), D98, J00, J01, J02, D05, J11
15. Explain respiratory distress syndrome (hyaline membrane disease). Add a note on 'pulmonary surfactant'.	521	633	D06(RS2), J11(RS2), N20(RS3), J06, D16

Contd...

Contd...

	GKPAL	SEMBU	
16. Timed vital capacity and its clinical significance	524	643	J17(RS3), J03, D14
17. Draw a labeled diagram showing FEV-1 in normal and restrictive conditions.	524	644	J07
18. The pulmonary function test done on a 50-year-old man with chronic cough and breathlessness showed a decrease in FEV1, normal FVC and decreased FEV1/FVC. a. Mention the type of respiratory disorder. b. Define dynamic lung volumes and capacities. c. Explain the utility of flow volume curve in the diagnosis of respiratory disorders.	524	643	J21(RS4)
Short Answers			
1. Name two muscles each of: (a) Normal respiration; (b) Forced inspiration.	509	631	D10(RS2)
2. What are accessory muscles of inspiration? Name them.	510	631	J05
3. Name the expiratory muscles.	510	631	D03
4. What is normal intrapleural pressure? What is its significance? Draw a labeled graph to depict the intrapleural pressure changes during quiet respiration.	510	634	D98, D10
5. Transpulmonary pressure.	512	635	J98
6. Explain the mechanism of ventilation during quite breathing.	513	632	J13
7. Mention any four lung volumes and its normal values.	514	638	D99
8. Tidal volume.	514	638	J18(RS3)
9. Define tidal volume and residual volume. Give their normal values.	514	638	J12(RS3)
10. Define the following giving their normal values: (a) Inspiratory reserve volume; (b) Vital capacity.	514	638,639	D01, D04
11. Define 'tidal volume' and 'anatomical dead space'. Give normal values.	514	638	D13
12. Draw and label different lung volumes and capacities.	514	638	D07

Contd...

PHYSIOLOGY

Contd...

	GKPAL	SEMBU	
13. Define residual volume (RV) and functional residual capacity (FRC) and give their normal values.	515	639	J21(RS4), D09, J14
14. Functional residual capacity (normal value and importance).	515	639	J11(RS2), D13(RS3), J15(RS3), J98, J08
15. Define vital capacity. Give its normal value. Name two physiological conditions where it is decreased.	515	639	D18(RS3), D99, J04, J15
16. Define: (i) Vital capacity; (ii) Timed vital capacity.	515,524	639,643	D98
17. What is lung compliance? What are its normal values? And in what conditions it is variable.	516	635	D12(RS3), J09, D11
18. Give the source, chemical nature and functions of pulmonary surfactant.	520	633	J08(RS2), D14(RS3), D99, D12
19. Explain respiratory distress syndrome (hyaline membrane disease) with its causes in adults and infants?	521	633	J00, D00, D01, D02, D04, D08
20. Explain factors affecting airway resistance.	522	637	D07, D14
21. Timed vital capacity and its importance.	524	643	D06, J13, D16
22. Forced expiratory volume (FEV_1)—clinical importance.	524	643	J14(RS3), J98
23. Maximal midexpiratory flow rate (MMEFR).	525	—	J06
24. Work of breathing.	525	637	J06

CHAPTER 67: PULMONARY VENTILATION

Short Essays

1. Dead space (definition, types, measurement).	530	647	D08(RS2)
2. What is anatomical and physiological dead space? Describe a method to determine anatomical dead space.	530	647	D10
3. Physiological dead space.	531	647	D18(RS3)

Contd...

PHYSIOLOGY

Contd...

	GKPAL	SEMBU	
4. Differentiate anatomical and physiological dead space. Describe one method to measure anatomical dead space.	531	647	D00
Short Answers			
1. What is the difference between anatomical and physiological dead space?	—	647	D10(RS2)
2. Define "dead space" air and give its importance. Give its normal value.	530	647	J11(RS2), D19(RS3), J04, J06
3. What are the types of dead space? Give their normal values.	530	647	J15
4. Physiological dead space.	531	647	D05(RS2), D15(RS3)
5. How is alveolar ventilation calculated? Give the formula.	532	647	D15
6. Calculate alveolar ventilation at a respiratory rate of 12 per minute, tidal volume of 400 mL and dead space air of 100 mL and comment.	532	647	J05

CHAPTER 68: PULMONARY CIRCULATION AND VENTILATION-PERFUSION RATIO

Short Essays			
1. Describe peculiarities (characteristic features) of pulmonary circulation.	536	628	D08, D09
2. Define and give examples of ventilation-perfusion ratio.	539	648	D07(RS2), D10(RS2)
Short Answers			
1. Mention the peculiarities of pulmonary circulation.	536	628	J21(RS4)
2. What is pulmonary edema? Name one condition where it is seen.	538	678	J16(RS3)
3. Increase of which capillary pressure in pulmonary circulation leads to pulmonary edema and explain the reasons.	538	678	J09
4. Ventilation-perfusion ratio and its normal value and significance.	539	648	D12(RS3), D17(RS3), J19(RS3), D14

Contd...

PHYSIOLOGY

Contd...

	GKPAL	SEMBU	
CHAPTER 69: DIFFUSION AND GAS EXCHANGE IN LUNGS			
Long Essay			
1. Describe the factors affecting diffusion of gases at the alveolar capillary membrane. Explain how to determine the diffusion capacity of lungs.	544, 546	652	J10
Short Essays			
1. Oxygen uptake at lungs.	—	653	J13(RS3)
2. Describe the mechanism of gaseous exchange in the lungs.	543	652	J13
3. Describe the factors affecting diffusion of gases through alveolocapillary membrane.	544	652	J07(RS2)
Short Answers			
1. Explain alveolocapillary membrane (respiratory membrane) with a labeled diagram.	544	651	J01, J03, J04
2. What is alveolar capillary block syndrome?	545	—	J09(RS2)
3. Explain the term 'partial pressure' of a gas and draw a graph to show the value of PO_2 in the: (a) Atmosphere; (b) Alveoli; (c) Arterial blood; (d) Mixed venous blood.	545	653	J05(RS2)
4. Normal values for O_2 and CO_2 tensions in air, alveoli and blood.	545	653	J06(RS2)
5. Give in a tabular column PO_2 of atmospheric, inspired, alveolar and expired air.	545	653	J12
6. Give the normal partial pressure of oxygen and carbon dioxide in the arterial and venous blood.	545	653	J02
CHAPTER 70: OXYGEN TRANSPORT			
Long Essays			
1. Explain oxygen transport from the lungs to the tissues. Add a note on oxygen dissociation curve. Write a note on Bohr's effect.	547, 549, 553	657, 658, 659	D15(RS3), J16(RS3), D11
2. Describe oxygen transport in detail. Add a note on acclimatization.	547, 557	657,682	D19(RS3)
3. Describe oxygen dissociation curve and explain the factors that cause right shift and left shift of dissociation curve.	549, 552	658	D08

Contd...

Contd...

	GKPAL	SEMBU	
Short Essays			
1. Oxygen transport in the blood.	547	657	J99, J08, J11, D13
2. Describe oxygen dissociation curve with a labeled diagram and factors affecting it. Give the significance of its shape. What is P50?	549	658	D05(RS2), D06(RS2), J07(RS2), D10(RS2), D14(RS3), D16(RS3), J04, J14, D16
3. Bohr effect and Haldane effect.	553, 557	659,661	J15(RS3), J18(RS3)
Short Answers			
1. Give the normal content of oxygen and carbon dioxide in blood.	—	—	J04
2. Oxygen dissociation curve with a labeled diagram.	549	658	D08(RS2), J00
3. Define P50.	549	658	J12
4. What are the effects of 2,3-diphosphoglycerate on oxygen-hemoglobin dissociation curve?	551	659	J10
5. Explain the role of myoglobin in oxygen transport.	551	—	J10, D10
6. List the factors that cause the oxygen dissociation curve to shift to the left.	552	658	D12
7. Explain Bohr effect and its physiologic significance (role in oxygen transport).	553	659	J21(RS4), D16(RS3), D02, J06, D16

CHAPTER 71: CARBON DIOXIDE TRANSPORT

Long Essay			
1. Describe in detail the various methods of carbon dioxide transport in the blood. What is Haldane's effect?	555, 557	659	D11(RS3), D10
Short Essays			
1. Carbon dioxide transport in the blood.	555	659	J14(RS3), J98, D09

Contd...

Contd...

	GKPAL	SEMBU	
2. In which forms CO_2 is carried in blood? Describe chloride shift?	555,556	659	D08(RS2), J09(RS2), J12(RS3), D02, D04
3. Describe the carbon dioxide transport in the bicarbonate form.	556	659	D12
4. Draw 'carbon dioxide dissociation curve'. Explain 'Haldane effect'.	556	661	D12(RS3)
5. Chloride shift.	556	659	D09(RS2), J17(RS3), J10
Short Answers			
1. Give the volume of carbon dioxide transported in arterial and venous blood. What is the significance of arterial pCO_2?	—	657	J07(RS2)
2. Name the forms in which carbon dioxide is transported in blood. Give its content in arterial blood.	555	659	J15(RS3)
3. Chloride shift.	556	659	D18(RS3)
4. What is Hamburger's phenomenon and where is it taking place?	556	659	J08
5. What is Haldane's effect? Where is it taking place? How is it beneficial?	557	661	N20(RS3), J00, J01, J02, J03, J08, J12, J14, D15
CHAPTER 72: REGULATION OF RESPIRATION			
Long Essays			
1. Name the neural regulatory centers of respiration and explain their role in regulation. What is apneusis? Add a note on "Ondine's curse". Add a note on 'Hering-Breuer' reflex/add a note on periodic breathing/illustrate Cheyne-Stokes breathing.	559, 561, 590, 570, 589	662, 664, 665, 674, 675	F21(RS4), D05(RS2), J12(RS3), D16(RS3), J98, D01, J08, J09, J11, D12, D16
2. What are chemoreceptors? Describe the chemical control of respiration. Add a note on Cheyne-Stokes breathing.	563, 589	666, 675	D12(RS3), D99, J06
3. Give the normal tensions of respiratory gases in arterial and venous blood. Describe in detail chemical control of respiration.	563	666	J05

Contd...

Contd...

	GKPAL	SEMBU	
Short Essays			
1. Give the location of respiratory centers. Explain how muscular exercise alters respiration.	559	662	D03
2. Location and functions of centers of respiration.	559	662	D17(RS3)
3. Medullary respiratory centers.	559	662	J14(RS3)
4. Describe the chemical control of respiration.	563	666	J08(RS2), J11(RS2), D06
5. Chemoreceptors.	563	666	J99
6. Name the peripheral chemoreceptors. Where it is present. How it will regulate respiration.	563	667	J02
7. Explain Herring-Breur inflation reflex. What is its importance?	570	665	N20(RS3), D07
8. Cough reflex.	570	—	D08(RS2)
Short Answers			
1. What are the functions of pneumotaxic center?	560	664,665	J15
2. Explain the voluntary control of respiration.	571	662	D09
3. List any four afferents that stimulate respiratory center.	571	665	D98
4. Explain the chemical control of respiration	563	666	D13
5. Herring-Breuer reflexes.	569	665	J06(RS2), J11(RS2), J16(RS3), J12, J15
6. Explain Herring-Breuer inflation reflex.	569	665	D06(RS2)
7. What are 'J' receptors? How are they stimulated and their reflex effects?	558	665	D15
8. What is the importance of cough reflex?	570	—	J11
Multiple Choice Questions			
1. The central chemoreceptors are present in: a. The carotid and aortic bodies b. **The floor of the IV ventricles in medulla** c. The arch of the aorta d. The carotid sinus	567	666	J21(RS4)

Contd...

PHYSIOLOGY

Contd...

	GKPAL	SEMBU	
CHAPTER 73: PHYSIOLOGICAL CHANGES AT HIGH ALTITUDE			
Long Essay			
1. Describe the mechanism of acclamatization to high altitudes.	575	682	J99
Short Essays			
1. List the effects of hypoxia at high altitude on body, specifying the mechanism for the change.	574	672	D98
2. Describe changes that occur during acclimatization to high altitude (low PO_2).	575	682	D15(RS3), J00, J08, J11, D11
Short Answers			
1. List four changes during acclimatization to high altitude.	575	682	J04
2. Acute mountain sickness.	576	681	J10(RS2)
CHAPTER 74: HYPOXIA, CYANOSIS AND OXYGEN THERAPY			
Long Essay			
1. Define hypoxia. Classify hypoxias and explain the features seen in the different types of hypoxia.	578	670	J09(RS2), D13(RS3)
Short Essays			
1. Classify and explain 'hypoxia". Give examples for each type. Mention distinguishing features of each type of hypoxia. Explain the role of oxygen treatment in the different types of hypoxia.	578	670	J06(RS2), D06(RS2), D09(RS2), D10(RS2), D12(RS3), J18(RS3), J02, D02, D04, J15
2. Define and classify hypoxia. Explain their causes and treatment.	578	670	F21(RS4)
3. Classify hypoxia. Explain any two of them.	578	670	J17(RS3)
4. Describe the causes and blood gas status of any type of hypoxia.	578	670	J07
5. Cyanosis.	580	676	J10(RS2), J15(RS3)
6. Oxygen therapy.	582	672	J09(RS2)

Contd...

Contd...

	GKPAL	SEMBU	
7. In which type of hypoxia oxygen therapy is most helpful? What are the effects of excess oxygen administration (oxygen toxicity)?	582	672	D15

Short Answers

1. Classify hypoxia (anoxia). Give example for each one of them.	578	670	J10(RS2), J00, J01, J14
2. Define hypoxia. Explain histotoxic hypoxia.	578	670	D07
3. Describe anemic hypoxia.	578	671	D15
4. What is 'stagnant hypoxia'? How does this type of hypoxia affect arterial PO_2 and oxygen content of blood?	579	671	D12
5. Two differences between hypoxic and histotoxic hypoxia.	580	671	D16
6. What is cyanosis? How is it produced? What are its types?	580	676	J06(RS2), D11(RS3), J18(RS3), D98, D00, J03, , D11
7. Central cyanosis.	581	—	J17(RS3)
8. Hyperbaric oxygen.	582	672	J10(RS2)

CHAPTER 75: HAZARDS OF DEEP SEA DIVING AND EFFECTS OF INCREASED BAROMETRIC PRESSURE

Short Essay

1. Caissons disease (decompression sickness)—causes, manifestation and treatment.	586	686	J16(RS3), D00, D02, D04, D15

Short Answers

1. What is dysbarism?	586	686	D14(RS3)
2. Caissons disease/decompression sickness.	586	686	D18(RS3), D06

CHAPTER 76: RESPIRATION IN ABNORMAL CONDITIONS AND ABNORMAL RESPIRATIONS

Short Essays

1. What is dyspnea, dyspneic index? In what conditions is dyspnea observed?	—	674	J09

Contd...

Contd...

	GKPAL	SEMBU	
2. Explain dyspnea and apnea with examples.	—	668,674	D17(RS3)
3. What is asphyxia? Explain its stages/ features (changes occurring).	588	673	D07(RS2), J01, D01, D11
4. Periodic breathing—define, its occurrence in various diseases.	589	674	D07(RS2), D14(RS3), J19(RS3)
Short Answers			
1. How do you differentiate Biot's breathing from Cheyne-Stokes breathing?	589,590	—	J10
2. Deglutition apnea.	676	669	J06
3. Apnea.	590	668	J18(RS3)
4. Name any four causes of apnea.	590	668	D98
5. Define dyspnea and apnea.	495, 590	668,674	J15
6. Dyspneic index and its normal value.	597	674	J14(RS3), N20(RS3), D14
7. Asphyxia and its effects.	588	673	D03, D06
8. Peptic breathing and its types with examples.	597	674	J08(RS2), D08(RS2), J00, J02, J11, J12
9. What is Cheyne-Stokes respiration? Name one condition where it is seen.	589	675	J14(RS3)
10. Explain the features of Biot's breathing. In what pathological conditions is it seen?	590	676	D10

CHAPTER 77: ARTIFICIAL VENTILATION AND CARDIOPULMONARY RESUSCITATION

Short Essay			
1. Artificial respiration—various method.	592	691	D11(RS3), D99, J12
Short Answers			
1. What is positive pressure breathing and its application?	592	692	D15
2. Artificial respiration—principles, methods.	592	691	D16(RS3), J13

Contd...

Contd...

	GKPAL	SEMBU	
CHAPTER 78: PULMONARY FUNCTION TESTS			
Long Essay			
1. Classify and briefly describe pulmonary functions tests in common use.	596	638	J07
Short Essay			
1. Lung function tests.	596	638	J08(RS2)
Short Answer			
1. List lung volumes and capacities.	597	638	J11

SECTION 7: GASTROINTESTINAL SYSTEM

PART A: INTRODUCTION TO GASTROINTESTINAL SYSTEM

CHAPTER 79: FUNCTIONAL ORGANIZATION OF GASTROINTESTINAL SYSTEM AND PRINCIPLES OF GASTROINTESTINAL REGULATIONS			
Short Essays			
1. Outline the role of mucus in different parts of gastrointestinal tract.	—	—	D03
2. Draw a cross section of the small intestine to show the various layers. State the role of enteric nervous system.	607	198,199	J05(RS2)
3. Name the components of the enteric nervous system and outline role of enteric nervous system in the gut.	609	199	J04
Short Answers			
1. Enteric nervous system.	609	199	J15(RS3)
2. Describe myenteric and Meissner's plexus of enteric nervous system.	609	199	D09
CHAPTER 80: GASTROINTESTINAL HORMONES			
Long Essay			
1. Give an account of gastrointestinal hormones with reference to site of production, regulation of secretion and function.	614	257,258	D08(RS2)
Short Essay			
1. How is gastrin liberated? What are its functions? Name factors that increase and inhibit its secretion.	614	257	J15(RS3), D03, J04

Contd...

Contd...

	GKPAL	SEMBU	
2. Name the gastrointestinal hormones. Describe the functions of cholecystokinin.	614	257, 259	D10
3. Cholecystokinin—pancreozymin.	614	259	D05(RS2), D15(RS3)
Short Answers			
1. Explain 'TROPHIC' action of a gastro-intestinal hormone.	614	—	J05
2. Enumerate the different (two) gastrointestinal hormones. List their functions.	614	258	J21(RS4), D99, D00, J03, D05, J06, D06
3. Gastrin (source, action, stimulants and inhibitors).	614	257	J07(RS2), J16(RS3), J19(RS3), J99, J05, D13
4. Secretin (source, action and stimulants).	615	259	D06(RS2), D13(RS3), J98, D98, J13, D16
5. Explain the role of secretin in regulation of bile secretion.	615	259	J11
6. Cholecystokinin/CCK-PZ (source, action and stimulants).	614	259	J12(RS3), J99, D14

PART B: GASTROINTESTINAL SECRETIONS

CHAPTER 81: PRINCIPLES OF GASTROINTESTINAL SECRETION AND SECRETION OF SALIVA

Long Essay

1. Describe the composition, functions and regulation of secretion of saliva.	621	203, 202, 205	J12
Short Essays			
1. Draw a diagram to show the pathway for salivary secretion when food is placed in the mouth (reflex salivation). Name four other stimuli that cause salivary secretion.	—	—	J05(RS2), D03

Contd...

Contd...

	GKPAL	SEMBU	
2. Saliva (composition and function and regulation).	620	203, 202, 205	D05(RS2), D09(RS2), J17(RS3), D12, J14
3. Explain the mechanism of salivary secretion and its regulation.	623,624	205	D13(RS3), D14(RS3), D02, D04, D05, D14, D16
4. Explain the conditioned and unconditioned reflexes which increase salivary juice secretion.	624	206	J08
Short Answers			
1. Saliva (components)—functions.	620	202	J10(RS2), D15(RS3), D17(RS3), J18(RS3), D98, J01, J02, D06, J13
2. Describe regulation of salivary secretion.	624	205	D07
3. What is conditioned salivary secretion?	624	206	J15(RS3)
CHAPTER 82: GASTRIC SECRETION			
Long Essay			
1. Describe the composition and functions of gastric juice. Describe various phases and regulation of gastric secretion with suitable experimental evidences.	628	210, 208, 213, 212	J01, D01, D04, D07, J10, J15
Short Essays			
1. What is achlorhydria? What complications does it lead to?	—	217	J08
2. Functions of stomach.	626	210	J07(RS2), D09(RS2), J17(RS3)
3. Functions of gastric juice secretion.	637	210	D17(RS3)
4. HCl acid secretion—mechanism with help of a diagram, regulation.	629	212	J12(RS3), D13(RS3), J14(RS3), J98, J99, J00, J03, D05, J11

Contd...

PHYSIOLOGY

Contd...

	GKPAL	SEMBU	
5. Regulation of gastric secretion.	631	212	J06(RS2), J07, J13
6. Explain the gastric phase of gastric juice secretion (experimental evidence).	632	215	D06(RS2), J14, D16
7. Pavlov's pouch.	632	212	D11
8. Paptic ulcer—etiology, pathophysiology and treatment (physiological basis, mechanism of action of drugs used).	636	217	D05(RS2), D16(RS3), D09, D10, J12
Short Answers			
1. Gastric mucosal barrier.	636	211	D06
2. Explain functions of gastric mucosa	627	211	D07
3. Name the different cell types of gastric mucosa. Mention the functions of each of them.	628	210	J02
4. Enumerate the functions of parietal cells.	628	210	D98
5. Composition and function of gastric juice.	628	210, 208	D11
6. Explain how gastrin acts on gastric juice secretion.	630	215	D10
7. What is the effect of vagotomy on stomach?	632	213,215	D05
8. What is the effect of sympathetic stimulation on stomach?	631	—	D05, J07
9. Explain the role of vagal stimulation of gastric juice secretion.	631	213, 215	J10
10. Explain sham feeding.	632	213	J01, J02
11. Gastric phase of gastric secretion.	632	215	J10(RS2) , D19(RS3)
12. What is 'peptic ulcer'? Mention two causes for it.	636	217	D15
13. Physiological basis of treatment of hyperacidity.	636	—	J10(RS2)
14. Describe how gastric acid secretion can be reduced to treat acid peptic ulcer.	644, 636	—	J11(RS2)
15. List the effects of gastrectomy.	638	—	D12
16. What are the sequelae after partial gastrectomy?	638	—	J09(RS2)

Contd...

Contd...

	GKPAL	SEMBU	
Multiple Choice Questions			
1. Chief cells of stomach secrete: a. HCl b. Mucus c. **Pepsinogen** d. Intrinsic factor	628	210	J21(RS4)

CHAPTER 83: PANCREATIC SECRETION

Long Essay			
1. Describe the composition, functions and regulation of secretion of pancreatic juice.	641	218, 219, 222	J00, D00
Short Essays			
1. Exocrine secretion of pancreas (pancreatic juice)—composition, mechanism, function (digestive), hormonal regulation of secretion.	641	218, 219, 222	J09(RS2), J12(RS3), D12(RS3), J13(RS3), J98, J02, D02, D04, D08, D09, J11, J12, D13, D14, D15
2. Proteolytic enzymes of pancreas.	641	219	J07(RS2), D11
Short Answers			
1. List the composition of pancreatic juice.	641	218	J21(RS4)
2. Pancreatic proteolytic enzymes—actions.	641	219	J99, D08, J14
3. Exocrine functions of pancreas.	642	219	D10(RS2)
4. Describe the actions of secretin and CCK-PZ on pancreatic secretion.	644	222, 223	D09
5. Enumerate pancreatic function tests.	646	224	D06

CHAPTER 84: PHYSIOLOGY OF LIVER, LIVER FUNCTION TESTS, AND PATHOPHYSIOLOGY OF JAUNDICE

Long Essay			
1. Differentiate between hemolytic and obstructive jaundice on the basis of relevant laboratory tests. Explain the differences in the results.	656	235,236	J05

Contd...

PHYSIOLOGY

Contd...

	GKPAL	SEMBU	
Short Essays			
1. Outline the formation, transport and excretion of bilirubin (bilirubin metabolism).	654	229, 230	J13(RS3)
2. What are the types of jaundice, their salient features and method of differentiation.	655	234,236	J11(RS2), D16(RS3)
3. Define jaundice. Mention the clinical features of obstructive jaundice.	655	234, 236	F21(RS4)
4. In a tabular column compare the urine tests used to differentiate pre- and post-hepatic jaundice. Explain the basis of their difference.	656	236	J05(RS2)
Short Answers			
1. List the functions of liver.	652	232	J05(RS2), D98, D99, J01, J02, D02, D06
2. Enumerate liver function tests.	653	234	J12
3. Bilirubin—source/mechanism of excretion.	654	229, 230	D06, D12
4. Jaundice (classify and one cause for each type).	655	234	J98, D08
5. Obstructive jaundice (blood changes).	656	236	J06, J13
6. Mention any two differences between obstructive and hemolytic jaundice giving the basis for the difference.	656	236	D98
7. State the differences between pre hepatic and post-hepatic jaundice.	656	236	D13

CHAPTER 85: BILIARY SECRETION

Short Essays			
1. Bile—components, functions, regulation of secretion. Name the effects of bile duct obstruction.	658	228, 231, 233	J06(RS2), J07(RS2), D15(RS3), J18(RS3), F21(RS4), D03, D07, J15
2. Compare and contrast liver and gall bladder bile. Mention the functions of bile	659,661	229	J21(RS4)
3. Explain the enterohepatic circulation. Give its importance.	659	227	J12(RS3)

Contd...

Contd...

	GKPAL	SEMBU	
4. What are the functions of bile? Explain the enterohepatic circulation of bile salts and its importance.	661,659	231, 227	D07(RS2), D10(RS2), D02, D04, D14
Short Answers			
1. Describe the functions of gallbladder.	—	233	J13(RS3), D09, J11
2. Bile—composition and functions.	658, 661	228, 231	J15(RS3), D19(RS3)
3. Compare hepatic and gallbladder bile.	659	229	J00, J05
4. Bile Salts (name and functions).	659	228, 231	J99, D99, J04, D08, D11, D15, D16
5. Enterohepatic circulation (of bile salts) and its functional importance.	659	227	D05(RS2), D13(RS3), J16(RS3), D00, D01, J02, J03, D04
6. List the function of bile.	659	233	J14(RS3), J00, D00, D01, D04, J07, D13, J14
7. Choleretic and cholagogues.	659	233, 234	D07(RS2), J10
8. Which substances are called cholagogues and what is their importance?	659	234	D08
9. List the effects of cholecystectomy.	660	237	J05(RS2)
CHAPTER 86: INTESTINAL SECRETION			
Short Essays			
1. Succus entericus—composition and functions.	663	265	D99, D11
2. Name the enzymes of succus entericus and their actions.	663	265	D11(RS3)
Short Answers			
1. Succus entericus.	663	265	J99
2. List enzymes produced by intestinal mucosa.	663	265	J04

Contd...

Contd...

	GKPAL	SEMBU	
CHAPTER 87: SECRETION OF LARGE INTESTINE			
Short Essays			
1. Functions of large intestine.	—	244	D06(RS2), D14(RS3), D99, J15
2. Name the bacteria in intestine. In which segment of gastrointestinal tract it is located? How does it help man?	667	256	J09
Short Answer			
1. Explain the functions of colon (large intestine).	—	244	J16(RS3), J00, J01, D07, J12, J13
CHAPTER 88: INTRODUCTION TO GASTROINTESTINAL MOTILITY			
Long Essay			
1. Explain the types of movements in different parts of gastrointestinal tract.	672	246, 249, 253	J13(RS3)
Short Answers			
1. Explain the genesis of peristalsis in small intestine.	672	253	D06(RS2)
2. Describe the initiation, progress and purpose of peristalsis in small intestine.	672	253	D11(RS3), D16(RS3)
3. What is migratory motor complex?	673	254	J09(RS2)
Multiple Choice Questions			
1. The following statements are true regarding peristalsis, *except*: a. Occurs at the rate of 2–25 cm/min b. **Parasympathetic stimulation inhibits peristalsis** c. It occurs only in one direction d. Apart from the GI tract it occurs in the bile ducts and ureters	673	—	J21(RS4)
CHAPTER 89: CHEWING AND DEGLUTITION			
Short Essays			
1. Deglutition reflex.	—	248	D06(RS2), J99

Contd...

Contd...

	GKPAL	SEMBU	
2. Deglutition—define, stages and mechanism with their regulation.	675	247	J06(RS2), D16(RS3), D18(RS3), J19(RS3), D06, D07
3. Name the phases of deglutition. Explain the pharyngeal (second) phase of deglutition. Add a note on achalasia cardia.	675	247, 249	J09(RS2), D09(RS2), J11(RS2), J14(RS3), D14(RS3), D15(RS3), J17(RS3), D98, D00, J03, D12, J13
4. Describe the esophageal phase of deglutition. What is achalasia cardia and its effect.	676	248, 249	D11(RS3)
Short Answers			
1. Centers of deglutition.	—	249	J06
2. Deglutition (swallowing).	675	247	D08(RS2), J98, J07
3. Write briefly on pharyngeal phase of deglutition.	676	247	D08
4. Enumerate four changes occurring during second stage of deglutition.	676	247	D14

CHAPTER 90: ESOPHAGEAL MOTILITY

	GKPAL	SEMBU	
Short Essay			
1. Achalasia cardia (cause and treatment).	679	249	F21(RS4), J06
Short Answers			
1. Role of lower esophageal sphincter.	679	248	J05
2. What is achalasia cardia (gastric)? What is it due to?	679	249	J10(RS2), J12(RS3), J04, J08, D08, D13, J15

Contd...

Contd...

	GKPAL	SEMBU	
CHAPTER 91: GASTRIC MOTILITY			
Short Essays			
1. Describe the movements of the stomach.	684	249	J06
2. What is gastric emptying time? Explain the factors which influence it.	685	250	J11(RS2), D99, J02, J05, J11, D13
3. Describe the causes and events in vomiting (emesis).	686	252	D11(RS3)
Short Answers			
1. What are the movements of stomach?	684	249	D11
2. Receptive relaxation—define, role in stomach.	684	250	J16(RS3), N20(RS3), J04
3. What is the effect of composition of chyme on gastric motility?	685	251	D05
4. What is the effect of fatty meals on stomach?	685	251	J07
Multiple Choice Questions			
1. Which of the following factor slows down gastric emptying: a. Vagal stimulation b. Gastrin c. Food rich in carbohydrate d. **Food rich in fat**	685	251	J21(RS4)
CHAPTER 92: SMALL INTESTINAL MOTILITY			
Short Essays			
1. Describe the different types of movements of small intestine.	690	253	D07(RS2), J16(RS3), D98, D01, J14, D16
2. Intestinal movements and slow wave.	690	253	J08(RS2)
Short Answers			
1. What are pendular movements? In which condition does it take place?	—	253	D07
2. What is myenteric reflex? What is its importance?	—	254	D02

Contd...

Contd...

	GKPAL	SEMBU	
3. Types of intestinal motility.	690	253	D05(RS2)
4. Small intestinal movements.	690	253	J19(RS3), J98, D11, J14
5. What is the importance of segmentation peristalsis in small intestine?	690	253	D08
6. Explain enterogastric reflex and its significance.	691	254	D11(RS3), D05, J10
7. What is paralytic ileus? What is its cause?	692	245	N20(RS3), D09

CHAPTER 93: MOTILITY OF LARGE INTESTINE

Short Essays

1. Describe the type of movements of large intestine and their functions.	694	254	J03, J10, D15
2. Mass peristalsis.	694	254	J18(RS3), D08
3. Describe the defecation reflex with illustration (mechanism of defecation in an adult).	695	255	F21(RS4), D12(RS3), D19(RS3), J05, J08

Short Answers

1. What is 'mass peristalsis'? What is its cause?	694	254	D13
2. What is gastrocolic reflex?	694	255	J07
3. Briefly describe the process of defecation (defecation reflex).	695	255	D10(RS2), D05
4. What is Hirschsprung disease?	696	245	J14(RS3)
5. What is megacolon and what are the causes and complications of this disease?	696	245	D07(RS2), J08, J09

PART C: DIGESTION AND ABSORPTION

CHAPTER 94: PRINCIPLES OF DIGESTION AND ABSORPTION

Long Essay

1. Describe in detail the digestion and absorption of fats. Add a note on steatorrhea.	700	266, 224	D17(RS3)

Contd...

PHYSIOLOGY

Contd...

	GKPAL	SEMBU	
Short Essays			
1. Chylomicron.	—	268	D19(RS3)
2. Describe the digestion and absorption of carbohydrates.	698	261	D12(RS3)
3. Describe process of digestion and absorption of proteins in GIT.	699	264	D19(RS3), D10
4. Explain the digestion and absorption of dietary fat.	700	266	D16(RS3), J18(RS3), D12, D15
Short Answers			
1. Name two substances absorbed mainly in lower small intestine. Give the role of any one.	—	—	J04
2. What are chylomicrons? How and where chylomicrons are formed and their functions?	—	268	D17(RS3), D08, D15
3. Give the site of absorption of: (a) Vitamin B12; (b) Iron in the gut.	701,702	241,75	J13
4. What is 'steatorrhea'? Mention any one cause for it. Give it's physiological basis.	700	224	D12(RS3), D10, D12, J13
5. What are micelles and how are they formed? What are its functions?	700	268	J11(RS2), D14(RS3)
6. Name the enzymes that help in triglyceride digestion.	700	267	J05
7. Enumerate the enzymes causing protein digestion.	699	265	J12
8. Name the important proteolytic enzymes and their mode of activation.	699	265	J11(RS2)

SECTION 8: RENAL SYSTEM

CHAPTER 95: GENERAL INTRODUCTION AND FUNCTIONAL ANATOMY OF KIDNEY

Short Essays			
1. Functions of kidney.	707	274	D18(RS3), J11
2. Endocrine functions of kidney.	708	411	J98

Contd...

Contd...

	GKPAL	SEMBU	
3. What is the length and diameter of proximal tubule of nephron? What the substances reabsorbed in this tubule?	709	277	J08
4. Juxtamedullary nephron.	711	275	J19(RS3)
5. Compare and contrast cortical and juxta-medullary nephrons.	711	276	F21(RS4)
6. Draw a diagram to show the structure of the renal filtration membrane. Explain the significance of each layer.	712	275	J04
7. Juxtaglomerular apparatus (formation, diagram, hormones secreted and functions).	714	280	J09(RS2), D10(RS2), J11(RS2), D13(RS3), J01, J03, J06, J09, J10, D11, J14, J15
8. Explain rennin-angiotensin mechanism.	715	281	D06(RS2)
9. What is renin? What is the stimulus for its production? How it will help in regulation of blood pressure?	715	281	J02
Short Answers			
1. Functions of proximal convoluted tubules.	—	277	J06
2. List the functions of kidney.	707	274	J05(RS2), D12(RS3)
3. Mention the non-excretory/extrarenal functions of kidney.	707	274	D01, D04, J12
4. How is the structure of proximal tubule of kidney related to its function?	709	—	D05
5. Draw a neat labeled diagram of a nephron.	709	276	J12(RS3), D06, J11, J14
6. Loop of Henle and its function.	710	277	J99
7. Name the synthetic functions of kidney.	707	274	D15
8. Explain functions of collecting ducts of nephron.	718	—	J07(RS2), D15(RS3)
9. Juxtamedullary nephron.	711	275	D18(RS3)
10. Draw a neat labeled diagram of the glomerular filtering membrane.	712	275	J09(RS2), D14

Contd...

Contd...

	GKPAL	SEMBU	
11. What is the physiologic role of mesangial cells?	714	280	J09(RS2)
12. Juxtaglomerular apparatus (draw a neat labeled diagram) and its functions.	714	280	J21(RS4), D09(RS2), D12(RS3), J14(RS3), J17(RS3), D19(RS3), D98, J99, D99, J07, J11
13. What is the important function of macula densa in distal tubule of nephron?	714	280	J09
14. Renin.	715	281	J98
15. Angiotensin II.	715	281	J99

Multiple Choice Questions

1. Angiotensin II causes all of the following, *except:* a. Simulation or thirst b. Increased ADH secretion c. **Vasodilation** d. Aldosterone secretion	715	281	J21(RS4)

CHAPTER 96: RENAL BLOOD FLOW

Short Essays

1. Describe the peculiarities (special features) of renal circulation. Explain the significance of one.	—	285	D18(RS3), D00, D11
2. Describe the hemodynamics of blood flow through the kidneys.	719	284,558	J06
3. Regulation of renal blood flow.	721	284, 558	J14(RS3)
4. Autoregulation of renal blood flow.	722	284, 558	J08(RS2), J13

Short Answers

1. List four special features (peculiarities) of renal circulation.	—	285	D03, J11, D12, D16
2. What is the cause of medullary hyperosmolarity in kidney?	719	—	D14

Contd...

Contd...

	GKPAL	SEMBU	
3. What is the functional significance of rich blood flow through renal cortex?	719	—	J07
4. What is the functional significance of slow blood flow through the renal medulla?	719	—	D05
5. Explain the role of `vasa recta' in renal function.	720	284	J05(RS2), D15(RS3), J08
6. Why is renal medulla very susceptible to hypoxic damage?	721	—	D07(RS2)
7. Define autoregulation of renal blood flow? What is its importance?	722	284, 558	D00

CHAPTER 97: GLOMERULAR FILTRATION

Short Essays

1. Define GFR. Explain the factors regulating the same.	724	286, 288	F21(RS4)
2. Tubuloglomerular feedback.	728	289	N20(RS3)

Short Answers

1. Describe the dynamics of glomerular filtration.	727	288	D14, D16
2. Calculation of net filtration pressure at glomerulus.	725	288	J13(RS3)
3. Give the formula to determine effective filtration pressure in glomerular capillaries and state the normal values. Explain the significance of any one.	725	288	J04
4. How much is the hydrostatic pressure in the glomerulus of malpighian body and what is its importance?	724	289	J08
5. Filtration coefficient.	725	288	J08(RS2)
6. Glomerular filtration rate (define, normal value, regulation, factors influencing, measurement).	725	286, 288	J07(RS2), D08(RS2), D09(RS2), J12(RS3), D12(RS3), D13(RS3), J15(RS3), D15(RS3), J16(RS3), J17(RS3), J19(RS3), J01, D01, D02, J03, D04, D09

Contd...

PHYSIOLOGY

Contd...

	GKPAL	SEMBU	
7. Filtration fraction—define and calculation.	726	287	J18(RS3), J98, D15
8. Role of angiotensin II in glomerular filtration rate.	728	288	D10(RS2)
9. Explain the tubuloglomerular feedback mechanism and explain the role of tubuloglomerular feedback in auto-regulation of glomerular filtration rate (GFR).	728	289	D19(RS3), J11

CHAPTER 98: TUBULAR FUNCTIONS

Long Essay

1. Describe the mechanism of formation of urine.	731	286	D06(RS2)

Short Essays

1. Na reabsorption in the renal tubule—sites and principles.	734	293	J21(RS4)
2. Explain the cause for splay in reabsorption of glucose by nephrons.	734	293, 294	F21(RS4)

Short Answers

1. Name the steps in formation of urine. Explain their significance.	731	286	J05
2. Define renal threshold. What is its value for glucose?	734	292	D05
3. What are the substances reabsorbed in the proximal convoluted tubule.	734	299	J12
4. Describe the renal tubular handling of sodium.	734	293	J12(RS3), J00
5. Sodium reabsorption by renal tubules (PCT).	734	293	J07(RS2), J13(RS3), J10, J13
6. Describe the reabsorption of water along renal tubules.	734	293	D00
7. Describe the reabsorption of glucose in the renal tubules with a labeled diagram. Define "TmG" and "renal threshold". Give the normal value for renal threshold and transport maximum for glucose. Name one substance which inhibits reabsorption.	736, 737	293,292	J11(RS2), D98, J00, D02, D03, D04, J07, D07, D13, J15

Contd...

Contd...

	GKPAL	SEMBU	
8. Glucose reabsorption curve in renal tubules.	737	293	D18(RS3)
9. What is meant by renal threshold for glucose and transport maximum of glucose (T_M for glucose)?	736	292	J19(RS3), J98, D01, D04, D12
10. Briefly describe the reabsorption of sodium in distal convoluted tubule.	740	293	D05
11. What is role of ADH in urine formation?	741	293	D14

CHAPTER 99: MECHANISMS OF URINE CONCENTRATION AND DILUTION

Long Essays

1. Describe the renal mechanisms of maintenance of normal specific gravity of urine.	746	295, 296	J06(RS2)
2. Discuss the mechanism of formation of concentrated urine. Add a note on diuresis/renal function test.	746, 758, 772	295,296	D07(RS2), J18(RS3), D19(RS3), N20(RS3)
3. Describe the role of countercurrent mechanism in kidney function.	747	296	J19(RS3)
4. Describe the countercurrent multiplier system. What is its role?	747	296	D12(RS3)

Short Essays

1. Describe the role of the kidney in water balance.	—	295	J13
2. Describe in detail how urine is concentrated in the kidney.	746	296	D14(RS3)
3. Countercurrent multiplier system in kidney.	747	296	D17(RS3)
4. Countercurrent mechanism and its importance.	747	296	J15(RS3), J98, D06, J09
5. Role of kidney tubule in countercurrent mechanism.	747	296	J14(RS3)

Short Answers

1. Briefly describe the countercurrent mechanism.	747	296	D05

Contd...

PHYSIOLOGY

Contd...

	GKPAL	SEMBU	
2. Which are called countercurrent multipliers in the nephron and what are their importance?	747	296	J08
3. Role of loop of Henle in urine concentration mechanism.	747	299	J08(RS2)
4. What happens to the tubular fluid in thick ascending segment?	748	300	J07
5. What happens to the tubular fluid in the collecting duct?	748	300	D05
6. The role of ascending limb in urine formation.	749	300	D16
7. Give the role of countercurrent exchangers in the kidneys.	748	297	J05
8. What is the role of vasa recta in countercurrent mechanism?	750	298	J16(RS3)

CHAPTER 100: REGULATION OF IONS AND WATER REABSORPTION IN KIDNEY

Short Answer

1. Name four hormones acting on renal tubules (influence urine formation).	752	292	D99

CHAPTER 101: WATER EXCRETION, DIURESIS, AND DIURETICS

Long Essay

1. Illustrate the mechanism of water reabsorption in different segments of nephron.	757	293	D11(RS3)

Short Essay

1. Compare water reabsorption in proximal and distal nephron.	—	—	D12
2. Mention the sites of water reabsorption in nephrons with its principle.	756	293	F21(RS4)
3. Diuresis.	758	323	J09(RS2)

Short Answers

1. Outline the differences in the reabsorption of water in PCT from that of DCT.	—		D13(RS3)
2. What is meant by facultative absorption of water and obligatory absorption of water? Where does it take place?	757	293	D01, D04, J06

Contd...

PHYSIOLOGY

Contd...

	GKPAL	SEMBU	
3. What is facultative reabsorption of water (in distal convoluted tubule) and the effect of its defect?	757	293	D15, D16
4. Explain how water is reabsorbed in collecting duct.	758	293	D10
5. Osmotic diuresis.	758	323	D05(RS2), D98, J14
6. Diuretics (Loop diuretics).	758	323	D16(RS3), N20(RS3)
Multiple Choice Questions			
1. The part of the nephron impermeable to water is: a. Proximal convoluted tubule b. Descending limb of loop of Henle c. **Ascending limb of loop of Henle** d. Distal convoluted tubule	757	293	J21(RS4)

CHAPTER 102: ACIDIFICATION OF URINE

Short Essays			
1. Acidification of urine—mechanism.	760	306	J21(RS4), D09(RS2), J17(RS3)
2. Describe the buffer systems of the kidney.	763	302	D09
3. Role of renal tubular buffers.	763	302	J13(RS3)
Short Answers			
1. Explain the mechanism of absorption of bicarbonate in the renal tubules.	761	302	D02, D07
2. Explain how bicarbonate ions are generated in the renal tubules.	761	302	J05(RS2)
3. How does renal tubule secrete ammonia? What is its role in acidification of urine?	760	307	J01
4. What are the substances synthesized and excreted in the collecting duct of nephron helping in increasing acidity of urine?	762	307	J08
5. Name the buffers of renal tubules.	763	307	D17(RS3)

Contd...

Contd...

	GKPAL	SEMBU	

CHAPTER 103: REGULATION OF VOLUME, COMPOSITION AND OSMOLALITY OF BODY FLUID COMPARTMENT

None

CHAPTER 104: KIDNEY FUNCTION TESTS AND RENAL FAILURE

Short Essays

	GKPAL	SEMBU	
1. Renal dialysis.	—	321	J10(RS2)
2. What is artificial kidney? Explain the physiological basis of artificial kidney. Give any two indications.	—	321	D06, D11
3. Describe/enumerate renal function tests. How is renal blood flow measured?	772	309,312	J06, D07
4. Postprandial alkaline tide.	773	305	N20(RS3)
5. Define renal plasma clearance of a substance. Give the formula for clearance and explain its utility in the study of renal functions.	775	311	D15

Short Answers

	GKPAL	SEMBU	
1. Nephrotic syndrome.	—	—	D08(RS2)
2. Artificial kidney—describe, principle, function, importance	—	321	J00, J02, J04, J09, J10
3. Inulin clearance test.	—	311	J15(RS3), J09
4. What is the normal value of inulin clearance? What is its significance?	—	311	D14(RS3), J14
5. What is creatinine clearance test? What is its significance?	—	311	D13
6. Explain why creatinine clearance is used to estimate glomerular filtration rate.	—	311	J05(RS2)
7. What is PAH clearance test? What is its significance?	—	311	D09
8. Explain urea clearance test.	—	312	D07
9. Alkaline tide.	773	—	J08(RS2), D08(RS2)
10. Name one substances used for measuring renal clearance and mention their significance.	775	311	J21(RS4)

Contd...

Contd...

	GKPAL	SEMBU	
11. How is a substance handled by the kidney if its 'clearance rate' is 160 mL per minute?	775	—	J13
12. Define plasma clearance in kidney.	775	311	D11
13. Define renal clearance. Give the normal value for PAHA and inulin clearance. What do they indicate?	775	311	D18(RS3), D00, J02, D02, J07
14. Dialysis.	778	321	N20(RS3)

CHAPTER 105: PHYSIOLOGY OF MICTURITION, AND BLADDER DYSFUNCTIONS

	GKPAL	SEMBU	
Long Essay			
1. Describe the nerve supply of the urinary bladder and the mechanism of micturition. What is cystometrogram?	779, 781	317, 319	D99, J02, D10
Short Essays			
1. Describe innervation of the urinary bladder with help of a diagram. Explain the process of micturition.	779, 781	317, 319	D03, J09
2. Draw a labeled diagram of innervation to urinary bladder. Explain how micturition is affected in spinal shock.	780, 782	317, 320	J05
3. Explain Laplace law. What is cysto-metrogram?	781	318, 319	D08
4. What is cystometrogram (pressure volume relationship in urinary bladder)? Draw a labeled diagram.	781	318,319	D05(RS2), D07(RS2), D17(RS3)
5. Mechanism and regulation of micturition.	781	319, 317	J16(RS3)
6. Describe micturition reflex. Write a note on automatic/atonic bladder.	781	319	J19(RS3), J12
7. Describe the spinal reflex arc for micturition, with a labeled diagram and explain two disorders of micturition.	781	320	D98
8. Automatic bladder.	—	320	J10(RS2)
Short Answers			
1. What is volume obligatoire?	—	—	D07(RS2), J11
2. Explain how the structure of the urinary bladder is suited to its function.	779	318	J05(RS2)

Contd...

Contd...

	GKPAL	SEMBU	
3. Parasympathetic innervation of urinary bladder.	779	317	J15(RS3)
4. Draw diagram to show nerve supply to urinary bladder and its sphincters.	780	317	D06(RS2), J09(RS2), D07
5. What changes take place as the urinary bladder gets filled with urine? Give reasons for the changes.	781	318	D12
6. What is "cystometrogram"? Name the physical law.	781	318, 319	D09(RS2), J10(RS2), J13(RS3), J17(RS3)
7. Draw a labeled diagram of pressure volume curve of urinary bladder or cystometrogram (pressure changes within urinary bladder as it is gradually filled).	781	319	J07(RS2), D01, J03, D04, D05, J07
8. Draw a diagram to show the pathway for micturition reflex.	781	320	D13(RS3)
9. Spastic neurogenic bladder.	782	320	D10(RS2), J14(RS3)
10. Atonic bladder.	—	319	D16

SECTION 9: ENDOCRINE PHYSIOLOGY

CHAPTER 106: INTRODUCTION TO ENDOCRINOLOGY

Short Essays

1. Radioimmunoassay.	792	—	D19(RS3)
2. Describe the neuroendocrine interrelationships.	788	340	J06

Short Answers

1. Define hormone. Explain characteristics of a hormone.	787	339	D09, J14
2. With an example, explain paracrine signaling of hormone.	790	339, 340	D14

CHAPTER 107: MECHANISMS OF HORMONE ACTION

Long Essays

1. Describe the mechanisms of hormonal action. Add a note feedback regulation of hormone secretion.	796, 793	343	D19(RS3)

Contd...

Contd...

	GKPAL	SEMBU	
2. With the help of suitable diagrams, describe the mechanisms of action of hormones through different system of second messengers.	799	345	D07(RS2)
Short Essays			
1. Explain the sequence of events involved in target cell response to hormonal action.	—	343	D11(RS3)
2. Cellular mechanism of action of peptide hormones.	—	344	D12(RS3)
3. Second messenger.	800	345	D19(RS3)
4. Explain the mechanism of action of steroid hormones.	806	346	J12
Short Answers			
1. Explain the importance of knowing the chemical nature of a hormone to a clinician.	—	344	D13
2. Mechanism of actions of polypeptide hormones.	—	345	D06
3. Role of cyclic GMP as a second messenger.	802	346, 345	D08(RS2)
4. Calmodulin.	805	345	J98
5. Explain the mechanism of action of steroid hormone on their target cells.	806	344, 346	D01, D04, J08

CHAPTER 108: HYPOTHALAMUS AND HYPOTHALAMO-PITUITARY AXIS

Short Essay			
1. Hypothalamo-hypophysial axis and its role in the regulation of anterior pituitary secretion.	811	347	J06(RS2), J01
Short Answer			
1. Inhibitory hormones of hypothalamus and their functions.	811	348	J07

Contd...

Contd...

	GKPAL	SEMBU	

CHAPTER 109: PITUITARY GLAND: THE ANTERIOR PITUITARY

Long Essay

	GKPAL	SEMBU	
1. Name the cells in the anterior pituitary gland and anterior pituitary hormones. Describe the mechanisms of action and regulation of growth hormone. Describe the functions of growth hormone and also the effects of abnormal secretion of growth hormone in children and adults (gigantism/acromegaly).	815, 816, 821	348,349	D08(RS2), D11(RS3), D14(RS3), D98, J00, J03, J05, D07, D10

Short Essays

	GKPAL	SEMBU	
1. What are the effects of hypophysectomy?	—	589	D09(RS2), J13(RS3)
2. List four factors that inhibit growth hormone secretion. Name other hormones regulating growth.	816	351	D06(RS2)
3. Functions of growth hormone.	818	349	F21(RS4), J17(RS3)
4. Disorders of growth hormone secretion.	821	355	D12(RS3)
5. Acromegaly.	821	355	J11(RS2), D16(RS3), J99, J07
6. Describe the effects of hypersecretion of growth hormone.	821	355	J09
7. Dwarfism.	821	356	D16(RS3)
8. What are the physiological effects of prolactin?	822	352, 472	J05
9. Describe the actions of TSH. How its secretion is regulated?	824	365	D03
10. List the gonadotropic hormones and their sources. Give their role in females.	827	351	D03
11. Give the source, target organs and actions of 'follicle stimulating hormone'.	827	351	D17(RS3)

Short Answers

	GKPAL	SEMBU	
1. What are somatomedins? What are their actions?	820	350	J06(RS2), D00
2. Acromegaly (cause, mechanism and clinical features with basis).	821	355	J21(RS4), J10(RS2), D13(RS3), J01, D03, D08

Contd...

PHYSIOLOGY

Contd...

	GKPAL	SEMBU	
3. Gigantism.	821	355	D18(RS3)
4. Dwarfism (pituitary dwarf).	821	356	D17(RS3), D14
5. Prolactin—functions.	822	352,472	D08(RS2), J19(RS3)
6. What are the effects of prolactin on breast development?	823	352,472	D16
7. Amenorrhea—galactorrhea syndrome.	824	—	N20(RS3)
8. Schematic diagram showing regulation of thyroid hormones.	825	366	J08(RS2)
9. List the functions of TSH.	825	365	D16
10. Gonadotropins—define and name them. Give the sources, target organs and actions.	827	351	D05(RS2), J04, J10, D13

CHAPTER 110: POSTERIOR PITUITARY

Long Essays

1. Describe the synthesis, transport, storage and functions of posterior pituitary hormones.	830	352	J11
2. Mention the hormones secreted by the posterior pituitary gland. Describe their actions and regulation. What is neuroendocrine reflex? Give one example.	830, 834	352	J07

Short Essays

1. Enumerate the hormones of posterior pituitary and explain the actions of any one.	830	352	J19(RS3)
2. Explain the regulation of secretion of antidiuretic hormone.	830	353	D17(RS3)
3. What are functions of ADH? What is the mechanism of action? Explain its role and its regulation.	833	353	J15
4. A patient comes with history of excessive drinking of water and passing of excess of colorless urine very frequently. Investigation revealed that the patient passed about 15 liters of urine in 24 hours. The urine was colorless, there was no sugar, blood or albumin in the urine. a. What is your diagnosis?	833	358	F21(RS4)

Contd...

Contd...

	GKPAL	SEMBU	
b. What is the cause for development of polyuria and polydipsia? c. In what other conditions polyuria occurs. d. How do you manage the condition?			
5. Diabetes insipidus—basis of any two features.	833	358	D05(RS2), N20(RS3)
6. Function of oxytocin.	834	353	J17(RS3)
7. Describe the milk ejection reflex.	834	354	J10(RS2), J12(RS3), D19(RS3), J00
8. Describe neuroendocrine reflexes with examples.	834	354	D15
Short Answers			
1. Explain why polyuria occurs in diabetes insipidus.	—	358	D13(RS3), D02
2. Antidiuretic hormone (vasopressin) and its action.	830	353	J10(RS2), D10(RS2), J99, J01, D01, D04
3. Explain how antidiuretic hormone acts on collecting duct.	833	353	J09
4. Diabetes insipidus (basis, lesion, features).	833	358	D18(RS3), D07
5. Mention the likely mode of development of diabetes insipidus and its resultant signs and symptoms.	833	358	J11(RS2)
6. Oxytocin.	834	353	D09(RS2), J13(RS3), J18(RS3)
7. Describe milk ejection reflex with diagram.	834	354	J07(RS2), D15(RS3), J05
8. Describe neuroendocrine reflex.	834	354	D00
9. Role of oxytocin in female reproduction/ parturition.	834	353	J03, J06

Contd...

PHYSIOLOGY

Contd...

	GKPAL	SEMBU	
CHAPTER 111: THYROID GLAND			
Long Essays			
1. Describe the steps in the biosynthesis, storage and release of thyroid hormones (thyroxine) and indicate the clinical application of this knowledge. Describe the regulation and functions of thyroid hormone. What is "Wolff Chaikoff" effect? Add a note on hypothyroidism/myxedema/cretinism. Indicate two sites where antithyroid drugs act and specify the substance at each.	838, 849	360, 365, 367, 369	D06(RS2), D10(RS2), D15(RS3), J16(RS3), D99, J02, D04, D08, J13
2. Describe the physiological effects of thyroid hormones (on general metabolism, cardiovascular system and central nervous system). Briefly explain the physiological basis of the features of hyperthyroidism.	844, 847	362, 366	D05, D16
Short Essays			
1. Describe the differences between 'pituitary dwarf' and 'thyroid dwarf'.	—	368	D02
2. Compare cretinism and dwarfism.	—	368	D18(RS3)
3. Describe the biosynthesis and functions of thyroxin.	838	360, 362	J06
4. Steps in thyroid hormone synthesis and their clinical applications.	838	360, 369	J15(RS3), N20(RS3)
5. Regulation/feedback control of thyroid hormone secretion.	843	365	J06(RS2), D16(RS3), D17(RS3)
6. Effects of thyroxine on body metabolism.	844	362	D08(RS2), D00, D01
7. Cardiovascular and CNS effects of thyroxine.	846, 845	363, 364	D07(RS2)
8. Explain the basis of three features of hyperthyroidism.	847	366	J05(RS2)
9. Hypothyroidism (effects of hyposecretion of thyroid hormone)—clinical features and their physiological basis.	848	367	J07(RS2), J14(RS3), J10

Contd...

Contd...

	GKPAL	SEMBU	
10. A woman aged 46 years consults her physician with history of swelling in the neck, weight gain, facial puffiness, swelling of the limbs and reduced appetite. Examination revealed enlarged thyroid gland, cold extremities, non-pitting edema and periorbital swelling. Thyroid function tests: T3—decreased, T4—decreased, TSH—increased. a. What is the probable diagnosis? b. What is the most common cause for the same? c. Explain the basis of non-pitting edema. d. Treatment of this case.	848	367	J21(RS4)
11. Myxedema (causes and features).	848	367	D12, D13, J15
12. What is cretinism? How can it be prevented?	850	367	J11
13. Enumerate thyroid function tests.	850	369	D09, J14
Short Answers			
1. What are the differences between pituitary dwarfism and cretinism?	—	368	D15(RS3), J11
2. Physiological basis of use of a drug in the treatment of thyrotoxicosis.	—	369	D07(RS2)
3. Explain the mechanism of action of thyroxine.	843	364	D10
4. Mechanism of increased BMR in hyperthyroidism.	848	362	D08(RS2)
5. Explain the cause of tachycardia in hyperthyroidism.	848	363	D14
6. List the features of Grave's disease.	848	366	J10(RS2)
7. Myxedema (clinical features).	849	367	J09(RS2), D09(RS2), J13(RS3), D00
8. Explain the skin changes occurring in hypothyroidism.	850	367	D16
9. Cretinism (clinical features).	850	367	J11(RS2), J12(RS3), J18(RS3), J98, J03, J07, J08

Contd...

Contd...

	GKPAL	SEMBU	
10. Thyroid function tests (describe any two).	850	369	J12(RS3), J17(RS3), D98, D98, J12

CHAPTER 112: ADRENAL GLAND: THE ADRENAL MEDULLA

Short Essays

1. Compare and contrast actions of epinephrine and norepinephrine.	—	408, 407	D09(RS2), J13(RS3), J03
2. Compare the effects of epinephrine and norepinephrine on heart and blood vessels.	—	407, 408	J05
3. Physiological basis of differences in cardiovascular effects of adrenaline and noradrenaline.	—	408	D08(RS2)
4. Describe the effect of any two hormones on stomach.	—	—	J07
5. Explain how the epinephrine secretion is regulated.	856	409	D13(RS3)
6. Enumerate the physiological actions of catecholamines.	856	408	D13

Short Answers

1. Name to adrenal medullary hormones.	856	406	J04
2. Name the catecholamines and give two actions.	861	406	J15
3. Explain 'flight or fight' reaction.	858	409	J09
4. What is pheochromocytoma? Which hormones increase in the blood circulation in this condition?	860	409	J11

CHAPTER 113: ADRENAL CORTEX

Long Essays

1. Enumerate the hormones secreted by adrenal cortex. Describe the actions, regulation of secretion of glucocorticoids. Add a note on Cushing's syndrome.	863, 868, 875	395, 397, 402	D12, D13

Contd...

Contd...

	GKPAL	SEMBU	
2. List adrenal gland hormones. What are steps in secretion of glucocorticoids? Write about the mechanism of action of glucocorticoids (corticosteroids) and about their functions. Add a note on Addison's disease.	868,877	395, 397, 404	F21(RS4), D16(RS3)
3. Describe the physiological actions and regulation of secretion of cortisol.	869	398,401	J19(RS3), D11
4. What are mineralocorticoids? What is their mode of action? Describe the regulation and functions of aldosterone. Add a note on Conn's syndrome.	878	395, 397, 404	D09(RS2), J13(RS3), D17(RS3), J10
Short Essays			
1. Functions of cortisol.	869	398	J17(RS3)
2. Describe the effects of cortisol on inflammation and allergy.	872	399,400	D16
3. Describe the actions of glucocorticoids/ cortisol during stress response.	875	400	J15(RS3), D05
4. Cushing's syndrome (causes and clinical features and their basis).	875	402	J06(RS2), J09(RS2), D11(RS3), J12(RS3), J14(RS3), J16(RS3), D00, D02, D09, J13, J14
5. Explain the basis of two features that are seen in hyperfunctioning of the adrenal cortex.	875	402	D06(RS2)
6. Enumerate the actions of aldosterone (mineralocorticoids). How is its secretion regulated?	878	395,397	J05(RS2), J16(RS3), D99, J00, J02, D04, J05, D10
Short Answers			
1. Diagram to show regulation of secretions of aldosterone.	—	398	D03
2. Name the zones of adrenal cortex and hormones secreted by them.	863	395	J03
3. Transcortin.	867	398	J98

Contd...

Contd...

	GKPAL	SEMBU	
4. Explain with an example "permissive action" of hormones.	870	399	J00, J01
5. Explain, why cortisol is not advised in patients with osteoporosis.	876	403	D07(RS2)
6. Describe the anti-inflammatory action of cortisol.	872	400	J12
7. Explain features of Cushing's syndrome.	875	402	J04, J10, J15
8. Addison disease (cause, clinical features and their physiological basis).	877	404	J21(RS4), J07(RS2), D07(RS2), J17(RS3), J01, J06, J09
9. What is the cause of hyperpigmentation in Addison's disease?	877	404	D16
10. Androgenital syndrome (clinical features).	878	405	D02, D06
11. Give typical findings in the adrenogenital syndrome in a post-pubertal woman.	878	405	D08
12. Mention the factors regulating secretion of aldosterone.	878	397	D01
13. Actions of aldosterone.	879	395	D16(RS3), J17(RS3), D06
14. Aldosterone escape.	879	397	D10(RS2), J11(RS2), J15(RS3), J98, J99, D14
15. Describe the effects of primary hyper-aldosteronism.	879	404	D11

CHAPTER 114: ENDOCRINE PANCREAS

Long Essays

1. Describe the physiological actions and regulation of secretion of insulin.	891,886	384, 386	D13(RS3)
2. Describe the physiological actions of insulin on carbohydrate metabolism. List the features of diabetes mellitus.	891,903	384, 390	D14

Short Essays

1. Regulation of insulin secretion.	886	386	D14(RS3)

Contd...

PHYSIOLOGY

Contd...

	GKPAL	SEMBU	
2. Factors that increases and decreases the insulin secretion.	886	386	J08(RS2)
3. Describe the mechanism of action of insulin.	888	385	D11
4. Mechanism of insulin action at cellular level.	888	385	D09(RS2), J13(RS3)
5. Principal actions of insulin.	891	384	J11(RS2), J12(RS3), D15(RS3), D15
6. Explain the action of insulin on carbohydrate metabolism.	891	384	J15(RS3)
7. Name the hyperglycemic hormones. Explain the mechanism of actions of any one of them.	895	390, 387	J01
8. Glucagon—sources, functions and regulation.	894	387	J08(RS2), D16(RS3), J98, D08, J09
Short Answers			
1. Human insulin.	885	383	J09(RS2), J99
2. Explain the regulation of insulin secretion.	886	386	D13
3. Describe the mechanism of action of insulin.	888	385	D09, J14
4. Name hypoglycemic actions of insulin.	891	384	D03, D12
5. Effects of insulin on glucose transporters.	890	384	D07(RS2)
6. List the features of hypoglycemia.	894	393	D12(RS3), D03
7. List the functions of glucagon.	894	387	J14(RS3), D00, J02, J15
8. Action of somatostatins.	896	388	D08

CHAPTER 115: BLOOD GLUCOSE HOMEOSTASIS AND PATHOPHYSIOLOGY OF DIABETES MELLITUS

Long Essay

1. Describe the endocrine regulation of blood glucose level.	899	389	J05(RS2)

Contd...

Contd...

	GKPAL	SEMBU	
Short Essays			
1. Hormonal regulation of blood glucose level.	899	389	D98, J06
2. Classify diabetes mellitus. Mention its clinical features and their physiological basis.	901	390	J21(RS4)
Short Answers			
1. Differences between diabetes mellitus and diabetes insipidus.	—	—	J14(RS3), J13
2. Renal glycosuria.	—	—	J99
3. Mention four hyperglycemic hormones that increase blood glucose level causing anti-insulin effect.	900	390	D10(RS2), D10
4. Diabetes mellitus.	901	390	D06
5. Explain why glycosuria occurs in diabetes mellitus.	903	391	J01
6. Explain why polyuria occurs in diabetes mellitus.	903	392	J03
7. Explain the basis of polyphagia in diabetes mellitus.	903	392	D09(RS2), J13(RS3)
Multiple Choice Questions			
1. All of the following causes hyperglycemia, *except:* a. Growth hormone b. Cortisol c. Catecholamines d. **Insulin**	903	384	J21(RS4)

CHAPTER 116: CALCIUM AND PHOSPHATE METABOLISM AND PHYSIOLOGY OF BONE

Long Essay			
1. What is the normal calcium level in blood? What are the functions of calcium ions in the body? Describe the role of different hormones in plasma calcium regulation. (endocrine regulation of serum calcium). Add a note on hypocalcemic tetany (clinical features). List two effects of hypercalcemia.	908, 907, 909	371, 372, 373, 374	D05(RS2), J07(RS2), D12(RS3), J18(RS3), D18(RS3), J99, D01, D09, J12, J14

Contd...

Contd...

	GKPAL	SEMBU	
Short Essay			
1. What is the normal blood calcium level? How it is maintained?	907, 909	371	D98
Short Answers			
1. List the functions of calcium in the body.	907	—	J02
2. Mention three hormones regulating blood calcium levels. State their mechanism of actions.	909	376	J15(RS3)
3. Explain the role of parathyroid hormone in calcium metabolism.	910	371	D08
4. What is the normal serum calcium level? List the hormones regulating it.	908, 909	375, 376	J11(RS2), J07, J11
CHAPTER 117: PARATHYROID GLAND, CALCITONIN AND VITAMIN D			
Long Essay			
1. Describe the physiological actions of parathyroid hormone. List the effects of parathyroidectomy.	918, 920	371, 372	N20(RS3)
Short Essays			
1. Regulation of parathormone secretion.	917	372	J07
2. Action of parathormone.	918	371	J14(RS3)
3. Describe the actions of parathormone. Name one antagonistic hormone. Describe the role of vitamin D in calcium metabolism.	918, 910	371	D99, J04, J08
4. Primary hyperparathyroidism.	920	374	J08(RS2)
5. What is tetany? What are causes, features and dangers of tetany. Describe signs of latent tetany.	920	373	D07, J15
6. Hypocalcemic tetany.	920	373	J06(RS2)
7. What is the normal serum calcium level? What are the features of tetany?	920	375, 373	D02
Short Answers			
1. What is latent tetany? Explain one clinical test to detect it.	—	373	J03
2. Four (functions) effects of parathormone.	918	371	D06, D10, D11
3. What are the features of hyperparathyroidism?	920	374	J12
4. What are the complications of hyperparathyroidism?	920	374	D07

Contd...

Contd...

	GKPAL	SEMBU	
5. Tetany (cause, physiological basis, clinical features).	920	373	J21(RS4), J09(RS2), J05, J09, D09, J14
6. List the features of hypocalcemic tetany.	920	373	D15(RS3)
Multiple Choice Questions			
1. Which of the following is not an action of parathyroid hormone? a. **Increases the renal absorption of phosphorus** b. Increases the production or vitamin D c. Mobilizes calcium from bone d. Increases the intestinal absorption of calcium	918	371	J21(RS4)

CHAPTER 118: ROLE OF CALCITONIN, VITAMIN D AND OTHER HORMONES IN CALCIUM METABOLISM AND BONE PHYSIOLOGY

Short Essays			
1. Calcitonin—source, target organs and actions.	923	374	J19(RS3)
2. 1,25-dihydroxy cholecalciferol.	924	371, 372, 381	J98
3. Give the source, target organs and actions of 'calcitriol'.	924	371, 372, 381	D13(RS3)
4. Physiological actions of vitamin D.	924	372	D14(RS3), D14
Short Answers			
1. Actions (on bone) and regulation of calcitonin secretions.	923	374	D03, J09, D16
2. Give, the source, target organs and the actions of calcitriol.	924	371	D13
3. Role of vitamin D in the prevention of osteoporosis.	924	372, 381	D08(RS2)

CHAPTER 119: PINEAL GLAND

None

Contd...

PHYSIOLOGY

Contd...

	GKPAL	SEMBU	
CHAPTER 120: LOCAL HORMONES			
Short Answers			
1. Prostaglandins.	933	413	J06
2. Atrial natriuretic factor/peptide (ANP)—action on kidney.	935	412	J08(RS2), J08

SECTION 10: REPRODUCTIVE SYSTEM

PART A: GENERAL REPRODUCTIVE PHYSIOLOGY

CHAPTER 121: SEX DIFFERENTIATION AND DEVELOPMENT, PUBERTY AND MENOPAUSE			
Short Essays			
1. Explain how sexual differentiation occurs in fetal life. Add a note on pseudohermaphroditism.	940, 944	426, 405	J13
2. Turner's syndrome.	943	14,15	J06(RS2)
Short Answers			
1. Explain what is Klinefelter's syndrome.	944	—	D13(RS3), D10
2. What is Turner's syndrome and how it is differentiated from Klinefelter's syndrome?	943, 944	14,15	D07
CHAPTER 122: PHYSIOLOGY OF PUBERTY AND MENOPAUSE			
Short Essays			
1. Describe the physiological changes that occur at the time of puberty in boys. (secondary sex characteristics in male) .	947	426	D14(RS3), D05
2. Physiology of puberty in females.	948	438	D08(RS2)
3. What is menopause? Give its basis and features.	950	456	J04
Short Answers			
1. Puberty.	947	438	J07(RS2)
2. Puberty and menarche.	947,948	438	D18(RS3)
3. List six secondary sexual characteristics in males.	948	426	D06(RS2)

Contd...

Contd...

	GKPAL	SEMBU	
4. Define menarche, menopause and amenorrhea and give timing of menarche and menopause.	948, 950	438, 453, 456	J05(RS2), J00

PART B: MALE REPRODUCTIVE PHYSIOLOGY

CHAPTER 123: MALE REPRODUCTIVE SYSTEM

Short Essays

1. Explain the functions of different types of cells in testis. What is 'capacitation' of sperms?	954	420, 460	D12
2. Sertoli cell and its role.	954	421	J09(RS2), D11(RS3)
3. Describe the blood-testis barrier.	954	422	D19(RS3), N20(RS3), D14

Short Answers

1. What is the importance of countercurrent exchange of temperature in the blood vessels supplying the testes.	952	425	J11
2. Sertoli cells—location and functions.	954	421	J05(RS2), D17(RS3), D19(RS3), D02, J11
3. Blood-testis barrier and its importance.	954	422	D06, J11, J12
4. What are the functions of androgen binding protein?	955	422	D16
5. Write the role of epididymis, seminal vesicle and prostate in reproduction.	956	420,431	J15(RS3)

CHAPTER 124: SPERMATOGENESIS

Short Essay

1. Describe the spermatogenesis and list the factors regulating it. Mention factors causing male infertility.	959	423	J10(RS2), D16(RS3), J18(RS3), D18(RS3), J98, D99, J00, J02, J03, D04, J05, D11, D13

Contd...

PHYSIOLOGY

Contd...

	GKPAL	SEMBU	
Short Answers			
1. Mention the methods of cells division with examples. Where it takes place?	959	—	D99
2. What is meant by mitosis and meiosis? Where does it take place?	959	—	J02
3. What is spermiogenesis and spermiation?	959, 960	423	J11
4. Define and explain "capacitation" of sperms and give the normal sperm count.	960	460,433	D11(RS3), J12(RS3), J05
5. List the factors regulating spermatogenesis.	961	424	D06(RS2), D17(RS3), J08, D12, D15
6. Semen (composition).	962	433	J10(RS2), D12(RS3), D02, J10
7. Changes after bilateral vasectomy.	963	—	J12(RS3), J04

CHAPTER 125: TESTICULAR HORMONES AND TESTICULAR ABNORMALITIES

Short Essays			
1. Endocrine functions of testis.	965	425	D18(RS3)
2. Describe the source and actions of testosterone in fetal life and adult life (at puberty).	965	425, 426	J11(RS2), D12(RS3), J14(RS3), D03, J08, D09, J14, J15, D16
Short Answers			
1. Endocrine functions of testis.	965	425	J17(RS3), J06
2. Give the source and any three actions of testosterone in adult life.	965	425	J13
3. What are the functions of testosterone?	967	426	D07
4. Describe the role of testoterone in fetal life.	967	426	D05(RS2)
5. Functions of testicular androgens.	967	426	J07

Contd...

Contd...

	GKPAL	SEMBU	
6. Inhibin (functions).	968	424	D08(RS2), D09(RS2), D12(RS3), J13(RS3), D05
7. Cryptorchidism—its effects on testis and its correction.	969	428	J99, D05, D07, D15
Multiple Choice Questions			
1. Which of the following is the primary action of inhibin? a. Inhibit the secretion of prolactin b. Stimulate the synthesis of estradiol c. Simulate the secretion of thyroid stimulating hormone d. **Inhibit secretion of follicle stimulating hormone**	968	428	J21(RS4)

PART C: FEMALE REPRODUCTIVE PHYSIOLOGY

CHAPTER 126: FEMALE REPRODUCTIVE SYSTEM AND OOGENESIS

Long Essay			
1. What are the functions of ovary? How are the ovarian functions regulated?	973	439	J09(RS2)
Short Essay			
1. Briefly describe the process of oogenesis.	973	439	J07

CHAPTER 127: DEVELOPMENT OF OVARIAN FOLLICLE AND OVULATION

Short Essays			
1. Describe briefly the formation and functions of corpus luteum.	978	447	D99, J04, J11
2. Describe ovulation and its regulation. What are test (indicators) of ovulation.	980	454	J07(RS2), D05, D09, J14
3. Explain the indicators/different tests for ovulation.	981	455	D16(RS3), J18(RS3), D12
4. Name four tests to detect ovulation. Explain the basis of any two tests. Calculate the likely day of ovulation in a 32 day menstrual cycle.	981	455	D03

Contd...

PHYSIOLOGY

Contd...

	GKPAL	SEMBU	
Short Answers			
1. List the various stages in the development of ovarian follicle. Mention three tests of ovulation.	976, 981	446, 455	J05(RS2)
2. What is corpus luteum? How is corpus luteum formed? Mention its function.	978	447	D14(RS3), J18(RS3), J00, J02, D06, D08, D11, J13
3. Ovulation.	980	454	J10(RS2), D98
4. What is ovulation and which hormone is essential for ovulation?	980	454	J11
5. Tests for/indicators of ovulation.	981	454	D07(RS2), D17(RS3), J19(RS3), J00

CHAPTER 128: MENSTRUAL CYCLE AND MENSTRUAL DISORDERS

	GKPAL	SEMBU	
Long Essays			
1. Describe with neat diagram, the ovarian and endometrial changes during menstrual cycle. Explain their hormonal regulation.	984	446, 449, 451	J15(RS3)
2. Illustrate the ovarian, endometrial and hormonal changes in menstrual cycle. What is amenorrhea and when does it occur physiologically?	985	446, 449, 451, 453	D15
3. Describe the ovarian changes during normal menstrual cycle. Explain their normal basis. Mention the tests for detecting ovulation. What is its importance? Explain the mechanism of fertilization.	984, 981,	446, 454	D02, J09
4. Describe the phases and regulation of uterine endometrial cycle. Explain the role of different hormone in each phase. Add a note tests for ovulation.	984, 981	449, 451, 454	J21(RS4), J17(RS3), D00, J01
5. Explain the interplay between ovarian and hypothalamic—pituitary hormones for regulation of menstrual cycle.	986	450	J08(RS2)
6. Discuss in brief the hormonal control of menstrual cycle. What is menopause?	986, 950	450, 456	J06(RS2)

Contd...

Contd...

	GKPAL	SEMBU	
Short Essays			
1. Describe the ovarian changes during a menstrual cycle.	984	445	D06, J13, J15, D16
2. Follicular phase of menstrual cycle.	983	445	D12(RS3)
3. Describe the endometrial/uterine changes during menstrual cycle.	984	449	J11(RS2), J12(RS3), J14(RS3), D15(RS3), N20(RS3), J12
4. Discuss the endometrial changes and hormonal control of 'proliferative phase' of menstrual cycle.	984	449	D13
5. Describe the endometrial changes occurring in the secretory phase of the menstrual cycle. What is the hormonal basis for these changes?	984	450	D01
6. Illustrate the stages of follicular growth in an ovarian cycle	985	445	F21(RS4)
7. Describe the hormonal regulation of menstrual cycle.	986	450	D10
8. Describe the role of FSH and LH in regulation of ovarian cycle.	986	450	D08
9. Hormonal basis of endometrial changes during menstrual cycle.	986	449	D10(RS2)
10. What is amenorrhea? When does physiological amenorrhea takes place in the woman?	986	453	J11
Short Answers			
1. Anovulatory cycles.	—	452	D16(RS3)
2. Explain how 'endometrial biopsy' is used to assess fertility.	984	459	D05(RS2)
3. List hormones regulating menstrual cycle.	986	450	J08, D11
4. Explain LH surge (cause and effect).	986	447	J16(RS3), J15
5. Physiological amenorrhea.	987	—	J98
6. Explain the physiological basis of lactational amenorrhea.	987	—	D14

Contd...

Contd...

	GKPAL	SEMBU	

CHAPTER 129: OVARIAN HORMONES AND CONTROL OF OVARIAN FUNCTIONS AND APPLIED ASPECTS

Short Essays

1. Explain the actions/functions of estrogen.	991	441	D11(RS3), J12(RS3), J08
2. Hypothalamo-pituitary-gonadal axis in females.	994	—	D07(RS2)

Short Answers

1. List (four/three) functions of estrogen on female genital tract/mammary gland.	991	441	D06(RS2), D12, D14
2. Actions of progesterone on fallopian tube, myometrium and mammary glands.	993	443	J14(RS3)

PART D: PHYSIOLOGY OF CONCEPTION, PREGNANCY, LACTATION AND CONTRACEPTION

CHAPTER 130: PHYSIOLOGY OF COPULATION

Short Answer

1. Explain the mechanism of ejaculation of semen.	999	433	J09

CHAPTER 131: PREGNANCY AND PARTURITION

Short Essays

1. Pregnancy tests (immunological tests).	—	469	J09(RS2), D16(RS3), D18(RS3)
2. Describe the structures and (hormonal) functions of the placenta.	1004, 1007	466	F21(RS4), J16(RS3), D01
3. Describe the (hormonal) functions of the placenta.	1007	466	J16(RS3), D01
4. Human chorionic gonadotropin.	1007	467	J10(RS2)
5. Discuss the physiological changes during pregnancy.	1008	461	D08
6. Cardiorespiratory changes in mother during third trimester.	1009	463	J07(RS2)
7. Describe the maternal changes in cardiovascular system during pregnancy.	1009	463	D14
8. Explain the mechanism of parturition.	1011	464	J12

Contd...

Contd...

	GKPAL	SEMBU	
Short Answers			
1. Explain the physiological basis of any one test to investigate the cause of infertility in a male.	—	—	D13(RS3)
2. Tests for pregnancy (name two with physiological basis) (immunological tests)	—	469	J16(RS3), D98, J06, J07
3. Factors causing movements of sperms.	1002	727	J07(RS2)
4. Fetoplacental unit.	1006	468	D09(RS2), J13(RS3)
5. Infertility in female (physiological basis of any one test).	1006	—	D09(RS2), J13(RS3), J19(RS3)
6. List the functions of placenta.	1007	466	J19(RS3)
7. Placental hormones.	1007	467	J09(RS2), J17(RS3), J00, J09
8. Human chorionic gonadotropin (source, functions and clinical significance)	1007	467	J14(RS3), J98, J10, D12
9. What are the structures that produce human chorionic gonadotropins (hCG) and mention the functions of hCG	1007	467	D07
10. Draw a graph to show the hCG level throughout pregnancy.	1007	467	J05(RS2)
11. What are the functions of human chorionic somatotropin?	1008	467	D16
Multiple Choice Questions			
1. Capacitance of sperm takes place in: a. Seminiferous tubule b. Epididymis c. Uterus d. **Vas deferens**	1002	460	J21(RS4)

CHAPTER 132: PHYSIOLOGY OF BREAST DEVELOPMENT AND LACTATION

Long Essay			
1. Describe the role of different hormones in growth and development of breast. What is the role of prolactin and oxytocin in lactation.	1015, 1017	471	J08

Contd...

Contd...

	GKPAL	SEMBU	
Short Essays			
1. Explain the importance of breastfeeding in prolactin secretion.	1017	472	J10
2. Describe the hormonal control of breast development and lactation.	1015, 1017	471	D15(RS3), J01, D10
Short Answers			
1. Explain the effect of individual sex steroids on mammary gland development.	1015	471	D13(RS3)
2. Hormonal control of lactation (enlist and specify their role).	1017	471	D99, D04, D06, D09, J14, J15

CHAPTER 133: PHYSIOLOGY OF CONTRACEPTION

Short Essays			
1. Describe the role of hypothalamus as a target for anti-fertility agents.	—	—	J06
2. Discuss the neuroendocrinal basis for the use of oral contraceptives.	—	476	D06
3. Oral contraceptives—contraindications.	—	476	F21(RS4)
4. Explain the methods of contraception in male.	1019	478	D00, J02, D04
5. Intrauterine contraceptive devices.	1019	475	D14(RS3)
6. Explain the mechanism of action of oral contraceptive pills to prevent pregnancy.	1020	476	J03, J10
7. Explain the permanent methods of family planning.	1021	477	J11
Short Answers			
1. On a line diagram, indicate the 'safe period' in a 30-day menstrual cycle and give the significance of this knowledge.	—	—	D05(RS2)
2. List the methods of contraception in female.	1019	478	D13(RS3), J00, J13
3. Intrauterine contraceptive devices (IUCD) and their mechanism of action.	1019	475	D18(RS3), J99, D03
4. Explain the mechanism by which oral contraceptives prevent pregnancy.	1020	476	D06(RS2), J11(RS2), J12(RS3), D01, D04

Contd...

Contd...

	GKPAL	SEMBU	
5. Endocrine basis of use of oral contraceptives in female.	1020	476	J15
6. Safe method of family planning.	1021	474	J09(RS2), J06
7. Permanent method of contraception.	1021	477	J07

SECTION 11: NEUROPHYSIOLOGY

PART A: INTRODUCTION TO NEUROPHYSIOLOGY

CHAPTER 134: FUNCTIONAL ORGANIZATION OF NERVOUS SYSTEM

Short Essay

1. Name the glial cells. Describe their functions.	1027	714	D10

Short Answers

1. Draw a cross-section of the spinal cord and label the prominent structures.	—	744	D06
2. Name the types of neuroglia and mention their functions.	1027	714	D99, J00, D02, J03, D12, D16
3. Astrocytes.	1027	714	D09(RS2), J13(RS3), D13
4. Oligodendrocytes.	1027	715	J19(RS3)
5. Microglia.	1027	714	D13(RS3)

CHAPTER 135: SYNAPTIC TRANSMISSION IN CENTRAL NERVOUS SYSTEM

Long Essay

1. Describe the structure of a chemical synapse with a diagram and the steps involved in transmission across such a synapse. Explain any two properties of synapses.	1032, 1037	722, 723, 725	J08(RS2), D01

Short Essays

1. Compare the mechanism of pre-synaptic inhibition with that of post-synaptic inhibition, with diagrams.	—	724, 725	D99

Contd...

Contd...

	GKPAL	SEMBU	
2. Define and classify synapses. Explain the two properties of synapse (occlusion and subliminal fringe).	1031	721, 725	J08
3. Draw and label a synapse.	1032	722	J07
4. Explain the steps of synaptic transmission. Name any one inhibitory neurotransmitter substance.	1033	723, 724	J13
5. Explain EPSP and IPSP.	1035	723	D18(RS3), D14
6. List the properties of synapse. Explain any three properties of synapses.	1037	725	D02
7. Write a brief note on postsynaptic potential.	1037	723	J05
8. Describe the different types of inhibition at the synapse.	1037	724	D06, D16
9. Explain Renshaw cell inhibition.	1038	725	F21(RS4)
10. What are the types of summation and how are they demonstrated?	1039	726	D15
11. Summation and occlusion in synaptic transmission.	1039	726	J07(RS2)
12. Explain the differences between muscarinic and nicotinic actions of acetylcholine.	1040	729	D09, J14

Short Answers

	GKPAL	SEMBU	
1. Explain synaptic fatigue.	—	726	J09
2. Synapse.	1031	721	D98
3. What is synapse? Mention three types of synapses in nervous system.	1031	721	J11
4. What is IPSP and EPSP in the synapse?	1035	723	J11
5. Important features of EPSP.	1035	723	J14(RS3)
6. List four features of synaptic transmission.	1037	725	D03
7. List four properties of a synapse.	1037	725	D14
8. Synaptic delay.	1037	726	D16(RS3), J18(RS3)
9. Explain the role of synaptic inhibition.	1037	724	D06(RS2)

Contd...

Contd...

	GKPAL	SEMBU	
10. Explain Renshaw's cell inhibition.	1038	725	J10(RS2), D15(RS3), J18(RS3), J00, D01, J04, D04, D05, D11, D13
11. Explain presynaptic inhibition with a diagram.	1037	725	J04, J08, D09, J14
12. Different types of summation in neurons.	1039	726	J08(RS2)
13. Explain the property of synaptic occlusion.	1039	725	J12
14. Name the neurotransmitters in the CNS.	1040	728	J10(RS2)
15. Gamma aminobutyric acid (GABA).	1041	731	D12(RS3)

PART B: THE SENSORY SYSTEM

CHAPTER 136: INTRODUCTION TO SENSORY SYSTEM AND PHYSIOLOGY OF RECEPTORS

Long Essay

1. Classify sensory receptors. Give examples for each. Explain their properties.	1046	716	J11(RS2), D17(RS3), J04

Short Essays

1. Give the classification of receptors. Describe properties of receptors.	1046	716	D11, D12
2. Name the cutaneous receptors. How is receptor potential developed?	1046	717	J11
3. Generator potential.	1049	719	D98
4. Properties of sensory receptors.	1049	717	D12(RS3)
5. Explain adaptation of sensory receptors and its significance with examples.	1049	717	D05(RS2)
6. Explain the basis of: (a) Intensity discrimination; (b) Localization of stimulus.	1050	717	D06(RS2)
7. Weber Fechner law.	1050	719	D19(RS3)

Short Answers

1. Classify sensory receptors (axons) and their functions.	1046	716	D05(RS2), J06

Contd...

Contd...

	GKPAL	SEMBU	
2. Name three touch receptors. Enumerate three properties of them.	1046	717	J16(RS3)
3. Thermal receptors and their location.	1046	717	D06(RS2), J04, J07, D15
4. Pacinian corpuscle.	1047	717	J07(RS2), D98
5. Explain the mechanism and purpose of 'adaptation' observed in certain sensory 'receptors'.	1049	717	D19(RS3), D13
6. Weber Fechner's law.	1050	719	J11
7. Explain the "Muller's doctrine" of specific nerve energies.	1050	717	D08, J11
8. Law of projection.	1050	719	J11
9. What is Phantom limb? Explain law of projection.	1050	720	D09, J14
10. Phantom limb and its basis.	1050	720	D05(RS2), J11(RS2), J98, J02

CHAPTER 137: SENSORY COMMUNICATION TO SPINAL CORD

Short Essays

1. Epicritic and protopathic sensations.	—	—	J99
2. What are synthetic senses? Give examples.	—	—	J05

Short Answers

1. Define sensory unit and dermatome.	1052	778	J08
2. What is Bell-Magendie's law? What is the exception to this law?	1054	725	D16(RS3), D05, J11

CHAPTER 138: ASCENDING PATHWAYS

Long Essays

1. Describe the dorsal column tract and its functions. How its functions are affected in Brown Sequard's syndrome?	1058, 1087	753,763	J16(RS3)
2. Trace the pathway for touch sensation with the help of diagram. What are the effects of "Tabes dorsalis" on sensory functions?	1060, 1087	753, 763, 765	D11(RS3), J12(RS3)

Contd...

Contd...

	GKPAL	SEMBU	
Short Essays			
1. Name the sensory tracts and explain the origin, course and termination of ventral spinocerebellar tract.	1058	749, 750	J11
2. Describe the pathway of fine touch with a labeled diagram (dorsal column) from right hand. List other sensations carried by this pathway.	1058	753	J98, D99, D08
3. What is Rhomberg's sign and in what diseases this sign is positive?	1062	—	D07
Short Answers			
1. Explain the effects of unilateral lesion of 'dorsal nerve roots'.	—	—	D13
2. Explain the origin, course and functions of dorsal spinocerebellar tract.	—	750	D09, J14
3. Name the ascending tracts and sensations carried by them.	1058	749	J07
4. Name the tracts in posterior white column of spinal cord. What sensations are carried by these tracts?	1058	749	J11
5. Draw the diagram showing dorsal column lemniscal system.	1058	754	J08(RS2)
6. List the sensations carried by the dorsal column tract.	1058	749	J05(RS2)
7. Explain stereognosis.	1061	755	J10(RS2), D19(RS3), J02
8. Dissociated anesthesia (where it is seen).	1061	763	D07(RS2), N20(RS3)

CHAPTER 139: PHYSIOLOGY OF PAIN, ITCH AND TEMPERATURE

Long Essays			
1. Describe the pain pathway. Write important features of fast and slow pain.	1066	778,777	J14(RS3)
2. Trace the pathways for different types of pain. What are the endogenous pain inhibitory pathways? Write a note on visceral pain.	1066, 1068, 1070	778,780	D98

Contd...

Contd...

	GKPAL	SEMBU	
3. Draw a neat labeled diagram of 'slow pain' pathway from right lower limb. Explain 'descending analgesia system'.	1067, 1070	751,780	J19(RS3)
4. Draw diagram to show the somatic pain pathways from: (a) Limbs/Soma; (b) Face. Explain the endogenous analgesia system (four ways by which pain sensations can be blocked).	1066, 1074, 1070	751,780	J05(RS2), D03
5. Draw a neat labeled diagram of 'fast pain' pathway from left lower limb. Explain 'referred pain'.	1067, 1069	751, 777	D13(RS3)
Short Essays			
1. Compare fast pain with slow pain.	—	777	F21(RS4)
2. Pathways for fast and slow pain.	1066	751	D08(RS2)
3. Describe the neural mechanism of pain. Add a note on acupuncture analgesia.	1066	778	J06
4. Visceral pain.	1068	777	D98
5. Define 'referred pain'. Give any two examples of referred pain. Explain its physiological basis.	1068	777	J07(RS2), J10(RS2), J98, J00, J07, J12, J13, J15
6. Endogenous pain inhibiting system and its role.	1070	780	D07(RS2), J01, J02, D02, D04, J09
Short Answers			
1. Physiological basis of use of a drug in relieving inflammatory pain.	—	—	D08(RS2)
2. Briefly describe the differences between fast and slow pain.	—	777	D05
3. List four special features of visceral pain.	1068	777	D16
4. Referred pain.	1068	777	J06
5. Describe the mechanism of referred pain.	1069	777	J10
6. Dermatomal theory of referred pain.	1069	777	D07(RS2)
7. Name the endogenous opioid peptides. Mention their role.	1070	732	J13

Contd...

Contd...

	GKPAL	SEMBU	
Multiple Choice Questions			
1. Nociceptive stimuli are transmitted by: a. Pacinian corpuscle b. **Naked nerve endings** c. Merkel's disk d. Ruffini end organ	1065	717	J21(RS4)

CHAPTER 140: TRIGEMINAL SYSTEM

None

CHAPTER 141: THALAMUS

Long Essay			
1. Describe the nuclei, connections and functions of the thalamus with suitable diagrams. Add a note on phantom limb.	1076, 1050	786, 787, 789, 790	J07
Short Essays			
1. Describe the nuclei and functions of thalamus. Add a note on thalamic syndrome.	1076	786, 789, 790	J21(RS4), J06(RS2), J18(RS3), J19(RS3), N20(RS3), D16
2. Why thalamus is called the sensory relay station.	1080	789	F21(RS4)
3. Thalamic syndrome.	1081	790	J14(RS3)
Short Answer			
1. List the features of thalamic syndrome.	1081	790	D15(RS3), D18(RS3)

CHAPTER 142: SENSORY CORTEX

Short Essays			
1. Explain the location and functions of somatosensory area of cerebral cortex.	1083	828	D12
2. Somatosensory area I.	1084	828	D14(RS3)
Short Answer			
1. Mention the features of representation of the body in the sensory cortex (sensory homunculus).	1084	828	D01, D03, D04

Contd...

Contd...

	GKPAL	SEMBU	
CHAPTER 143: SENSORY ABNORMALITIES			
Short Essay			
1. Brown-Sequard syndrome.	1087	763	J09(RS2), J19(RS3), D06, J11
Short Answers			
1. Brown-Sequard syndrome—clinical features below the level of lesion.	1087	763	D14(RS3), J18(RS3)
2. Syringomyelia.	1087	755	J06
PART C: THE MOTOR SYSTEM			
CHAPTER 144: INTRODUCTION TO AND ORGANIZATION OF MOTOR SYSTEM			
None			
CHAPTER 145: SEGMENTAL ORGANIZATION OF MOTOR SYSTEM			
None			
CHAPTER 146: MUSCLE SPINDLE AND GOLGI TENDON ORGAN			
Long Essays			
1. Draw a neat labeled diagram of the muscle spindle. Explain how muscle tone is maintained in the body.	1099	843, 844	D09(RS2), J13(RS3)
2. What are the components of a monosynaptic reflex? Explain the role of muscle spindle in the regulation of muscle length.	1100	843	D05
Short Essay			
1. Describe the structure of muscle spindle and its functions.	1099	841, 843	J10(RS2), D16(RS3), D01
Short Answers			
1. Muscle spindle.	1099	841	D10(RS2)
2. Draw and label structure and innervation of muscle spindle.	1099	843	D06(RS2), D08
3. Draw and label Golgi Tendon organ. What are its functions?	1102	843	D09, J14

Contd...

Contd...

	GKPAL	SEMBU	
CHAPTER 147: SPINAL REFLEXES			
Long Essays			
1. Give the clinical classification of reflexes. Give examples for each. Draw a labeled diagram of spinal reflex arc. Explain how reflexes are useful in clinical examination.	1104	736, 738	D03
2. Define reflex action. Give different types of classifications of reflexes. Describe four important properties of reflexes.	1104	734	D11
Short Essays			
1. Draw the reflex arc for knee jerk. Explain the basis of: (a) Exaggerated knee jerk; (b) Loss of knee jerk.	—	734, 775	D00
2. Importance of clinical testing of muscle tone.	1106	844	D12(RS3)
3. Reciprocal innervation (neural circuit) and its functional importance.	1108	845	J01, J15
4. Describe the properties of polysynaptic reflexes.	1108	735	J05
5. Give the neural circuits for crossed extensor reflex, explain its functional importance.	—	850	J03
6. How is crossed extensor reflex elicited? Draw a diagram of its neural circuit and mention its purpose.	—	850, 741	D15
7. Name the superficial reflexes. What are the physiological conditions in which Babinski's sign is positive?	—	736,737	D07
8. Stretch reflex.	1104	736, 738	J07(RS2), J09(RS2), J15
9. Draw a diagram of reflex arc and classify reflexes.	1104	734,735	J11
10. Describe withdrawal reflex with a diagram and give its significance.	1107	735	J08(RS2)
11. Define muscle tone. Explain reflex regulation of muscle tone.	1106	846	J08

Contd...

Contd...

	GKPAL	SEMBU	
12. Define muscle tone. Explain its physiological basis. What is its clinical importance?	1106	846	D99, D00
13. Explain the effect of lesion of a: (a) Dorsal nerve root, (b) Upper motor neuron on muscle tone.	1106	191, 847	D17(RS3)
Short Answers			
1. Differentiate between superficial and deep reflexes.	—	—	J21(RS4), J15(RS3)
2. Draw the reflex arc for patellar tendon reflex.	—	844	J04, J06
3. Draw the reflex arc for knee jerk.	—	844	D05(RS2)
4. Explain reciprocal innervations.	—	740	D08
5. What lesions produce patellar clonus and ankle clonus?	—	738	D07
6. Draw the neural circuit for crossed extensor reflex.	—	741, 850	D13
7. Draw and label a muscle stretch reflex arc.	1104	844	D12
8. Inverse stretch reflex—describe, name the receptors, physiological basis, significance.	1106	845	J17(RS3), J05, J13
9. Define muscle tone. What is its clinical importance?	1106	844	J00
10. Explain what is withdrawal reflex.	1107	741	D10

CHAPTER 148: SUPRASPINAL CONTROL: THE DESCENDING PATHWAYS

Long Essay

1. Describe the origin, course, termination and function of corticospinal tract (pyramidal tract) with labeled diagrams. Describe the role of corticospinal pathways in control of posture and movement. List the effects of lesion of the tract in right internal capsule. Or What is hemiplegia and paraplegia? List the features of hemiplegia.	1112, 1119	755	J09(RS2), D15(RS3), D99, J05, J09, D09, J14

Contd...

Contd...

	GKPAL	SEMBU	
Short Essays			
1. Difference between upper motor neuron and lower motor neuron.	—	—	J99, J01
2. Describe the functions of extrapyramidal tracts.	—	758	D11
3. (Compare and contrast) tabulate differences between pyramidal and extrapyramidal tracts/systems.	—	756	F21(RS4), D09(RS2), J13(RS3)
4. Pyramidal tract.	1112	755	J18(RS3)
5. Corticospinal tracts - Draw and label, course, functions.	1112	755	N20(RS3), J10
6. Trace the pathway of rubrospinal tract and write its function.	1115	760	D07
7. In a tabular column compare the features of upper motor neuron lesions and lower motor neuron lesions.	1118	775	D06(RS2), J11(RS2), J16(RS3), J17(RS3), D19(RS3)
Short Answers			
1. Babinski sign—causes, significance.	—	737	J06(RS2), D11(RS3), J12(RS3), D19(RS3), J18(RS3), J98, D01, D04, J10, J12
2. Upper motor neuron.	—	847	D98
3. Mention four features of lesion to corticospinal fibers at right internal capsule level.	1114	817	J13
4. List the signs of the upper motor neuron lesion.	1114	775	D14(RS3), J00, D02, D11, J15
5. Enumerate the features of lower motor neuron paralysis.	1118	775	N20(RS3)
6. What is hemiplegia and involvement of which motor tract leads to hemiplegia?	1119	775	D07

Contd...

Contd...

	GKPAL	SEMBU	
CHAPTER 149: REGULATION OF MUSCLE TONE, POSTURE AND MOVEMENT: SPINAL, MEDULLARY, MIDBRAIN AND CORTICAL INTEGRATION			
Long Essays			
1. Describe the role of spinal cord and medulla in the control of movement and posture.	1124, 1126	846	D08(RS2)
2. Describe the immediate effects of complete transection of the spinal cord at midthoracic level and explain the basis of these effects.	1124	761	D06(RS2)
3. Describe the neurological changes that are seen 4 weeks after complete transection of the spinal cord at L-1 level.	1124	762	D05(RS2)
Short Essays			
1. Explain with the help of a diagram, clinical features (sensory and motor changes) in a hemisection of spinal cord.	—	763	J21(RS4), D00, J03, D08, D15
2. Tabulate the differences between classical decerebration and ischemic decerebration.	—	839	D09(RS2), J13(RS3)
3. Complete transaction of the spinal cord.	1124	761	J17(RS3)
4. Stages and features of spinal shock.	1124	761	D16(RS3)
5. Describe the mass reflex and its basis.	1125	762	D05
6. Site of lesion and reflexes present in decerebrate cat.	1126	840	J06(RS2)
7. Decerebrate rigidity—features and physiological basis/mechanism.	1126	840	D14(RS3), J12, D14
8. Describe the righting reflexes, their significance and neural level of integration.	1128	848	D15
Short Answers			
1. Describe the immediate effects of spinal transection.	1124	761	D05
2. Spinal shock and its features.	1124	761	J02, D06
3. Explains mass reflex and its basis.	1125	762	J06(RS2), D06(RS2), J08(RS2), J04

Contd...

Contd...

	GKPAL	SEMBU	
4. Decorticate rigidity.	1130	839	J08(RS2)
5. Describe the functions and the features of primary motor area.	1130	823	J09
6. Describe the representation on motor homunculus.	1131	825	J05(RS2), D17(RS3), J04

CHAPTER 150: BASAL GANGLIA

Long Essay

1. Describe the nuclei, connections and functions of the basal ganglia. Mention the features of basal ganglia lesion. Add a note on its disorders/Parkinson's disease (pathophysiology, clinical features, physiological principles of treatment).	1134	814,817	J21(RS4), J10(RS2), J18(RS3), D18(RS3), D19(RS3), J98, J01, J02, D04, D06, D12, D16

Short Essays

1. Basal ganglia—enumerate structures forming, principal connections and functions.	1134	814	F21(RS4), J11(RS2), J19(RS3), D07
2. Nigrostriatal pathway.	1135	817	D12(RS3)
3. List four features of basal ganglia disease and explain the basis of any one.	1137	817	J05(RS2)
4. Write a short essay on Parkinsonism (cause, clinical features and treatment).	1137	817	J09(RS2), D15(RS3), D01
5. Describe the features and physiological basis of Parkinsonism.	1137	817	D13

Short Answers

1. Differentiate between lead pipe rigidity and cog-wheel rigidity.	—	—	J10
2. Paralysis agitance (Parkinsonism) and its features.	1137	817	D98, J99, D99, J07
3. Explain what is 'lead-pipe' and 'clasp-knife' rigidity in what pathological conditions are they found.	1138	818	D10
4. Chorea.	1138	819	J07(RS2)

Contd...

PHYSIOLOGY

Contd...

	GKPAL	SEMBU	
CHAPTER 151: CEREBELLUM			
Long Essays			
1. Name the functional divisions of the cerebellum. Describe the structure, connections and functions of cerebellum. Mention two signs of cerebellar lesions.	1141	801, 812	J15(RS3), J99, J00, D02, J08
2. Describe the input, output, internal connections and functions of cerebellum. Add a note on clinical features seen in cerebellar dysfunction.	1140	801, 812	D14(RS3), D14, J15
3. Discuss how cerebellum controls motor activity. Add a note on tests of cerebellar function.	1144, 1146	811, 813	J13
4. List the features of cerebellar disorder. Describe the role of cerebellum in the control of motor functions.	1144, 1146,	811, 812	D07(RS2)
Short Essays			
1. Functions of spinocerebellum.	1141	809	D08(RS2)
2. Name cerebellar nuclei. How is dentate nucleus connected to motor area of cerebral cortex?	1141	804	D07
3. Describe briefly important connections and functions of neocerebellum (cerebro-cerebellum).	1141	803	D13(RS3)
4. Functions of cerebellum.	1144	812	D15(RS3)
5. Explain the role of cerebellum in co-ordination of movements.	1145	811	D10
6. Define muscle tone. Describe supraspinal control of muscle tone.	1145	846, 847	J04
7. List four features of cerebellar disorders and explain any one.	1146	812	D05(RS2)
8. Describe the characteristic features of cerebellar lesion.	1146	812	J12(RS3), D17(RS3), D09, J14
Short Answers			
1. Explain the functions of flocculonodular lobe.	1141	806	D08
2. Draw the main connections of neocerebellum with cerebral cortex.	1143	803	J16(RS3)

Contd...

Contd...

	GKPAL	SEMBU	
3. Alpha-gamma colinkage.	1145	846	D08(RS2)
4. How length servomechanism operates to maintain muscle length.	1145	812	F21(RS4)
5. Name four features of cerebellar lesions.	1146	812	D03
6. Adiadochokinesia.	1146	813	J98
Multiple Choice Questions			
1. Unconscious kinesthetic sensations are earned by: a. **Anterior spinocerebellar tract** b. Anterior spinothalamic tract c. Lateral spinothalamic tract d. Posterior columns	1142	808	J21(RS4)

CHAPTER 152: VESTIBULAR APPARATUS

Short Essays

1. Vestibular apparatus and its functions.	1148	851	J08(RS2), D98, J03
2. Write briefly on otolith organs.	1149	853	D10(RS2), D13
3. Name the receptors and functions of semicircular canals.	1151	852	D17(RS3), D18(RS3)
Short Answers			
1. Enumerate any three functions of vestibular apparatus.	1148	855	J16(RS3)
2. Otolith organs.	1149	853	D18(RS3)
3. Enumerate the functions of semicircular canals, utricle and saccule.	1151	855	D08
4. What is vestibulo-occular reflex?	1152	857	J05
5. Post-rotatory nystagmus.	1153	857	D12(RS3)

PART D: HYPOTHALAMUS, EEG AND SLEEP; LIMBIC FUNCTIONS AND HIGHER FUNCTIONS OF BRAIN AND CEREBROSPINAL FLUID

CHAPTER 153: FUNCTIONS OF HYPOTHALAMUS

Long Essays

1. Describe the various nuclei and functions of hypothalamus. Describe the regulation of food and water intake (role of hypothalamus in the perception of hunger and thirst).	1156	793, 794, 797, 798	D00, D08, J12

Contd...

PHYSIOLOGY

Contd...

	GKPAL	SEMBU	
2. Describe the principal connections and functions of hypothalamus.	1157	794	D12(RS3), D13
3. Describe any four functions of hypothalamus. Add a note on anorexia nervosa and hypothalamic obesity.	1157, 1161	794,797	J17(RS3)
Short Essays			
1. Describe the functions of hypothalamus.	1157	794	D09(RS2), J13(RS3), D16(RS3), J06, J07
2. Enumerate the functions of hypothalamus. Describe functions of hypothalamus/in the regulation of (a) Food intake; (b) Water intake.	1157	794	D98, J02, D04, J08
3. Explain the role of hypothalamus as an endocrine organ.	1157	794	D13(RS3)
4. Explain how hypothalamus controls secretion of pituitary gland (mode of hypothalamic regulation of pituitary hormones).	1157	794	D15
5. Describe the role of hypothalamus in regulation of temperature.	1158	797	D07(RS2), J11(RS2)
6. Role of hypothalamus in regulation of food intake.	1158	797	J15(RS3)
7. Regulation of water balance by hypothalamus.	1160	798	J14(RS3)
Short Answers			
1. List any four functions of hypothalamus.	1157	794	D99
2. Circardian rhythm.	1157	800	D10(RS2), D19(RS3), J99
3. Name two areas in hypothalamus which control body temperature.	1158	797	D00
4. Role of hypothalamus in hunger.	1158	797	J06(RS2)
5. Name the centers that regulate feeding behavior.	1158	797	D12
6. What are the locations of osmoreceptors and their functions?	1160	798	D15

Contd...

PHYSIOLOGY

Contd...

	GKPAL	SEMBU	
Multiple Choice Questions			
1. The satiety center is located in which portion of hypothalamus: a. Lateral nucleus b. Preoptlc area c. **Ventromedlal hypothalamus** d. Dorsomedial hypothalamus	1158	797	J21(RS4)

CHAPTER 154: PHYSIOLOGY OF RETICULAR ACTIVATING SYSTEM

Long Essays			
1. Describe the nuclei and functions of reticular formation.	1163	836	D07, D13
2. Explain the organization and functions of ascending reticular activating system of brain.	1164	836	D12
Short Essay			
1. Describe the functions of reticular activating system.	1163	836	D10
Short Answer			
1. Ascending reticular activating system.	1164	836	J06, J07

CHAPTER 155: ELECTROENCEPHALOGRAM AND SLEEP

Short Essays			
1. What is EEG? Discuss the neurophysiologic basis of EEG? What are its normal waves? What is alpha block? Or List the changes in EEG during different stages of sleep?	1166	860,861, 863	D11(RS3), J12(RS3), J16(RS3), J00, D00, J01, J03, J06, J09
2. Define sleep. Describe the genesis of NREM sleep.	1167	862,863	D09, J14
3. What are the stages of sleep? Write a brief note on REM sleep (mechanisms and features).	1168	863,864	D05, D14, D15
4. Stages of slow wave sleep.	1168	863	J06(RS2)
5. Control mechanisms of slow wave sleep.	1169	865	N20(RS3)
6. Compare REM and non-REM sleep.	1170	863	D98
Short Answers			
1. Electroencephalogram (EEG).	1166	860	J18(RS3)

Contd...

Contd...

	GKPAL	SEMBU	
2. Describe the various types of rhythms/waves that make up the electroencephalogram.	1166	860	D19(RS3), D10
3. Write a brief note on alpha block.	1167	861	J07(RS2), D05
4. Define sleep. Explain the characteristic features of REM sleep.	1167	862, 864	J98, J08
5. Explain the features of non-rapid eye movement (NREM) sleep.	1168	863	J12
6. EEG changes in non-REM sleep.	1168	863,864	J14(RS3)
7. Changes during slow wave sleep.	1168	863,864	D14(RS3)
8. Compare and contrast between REM and NREM (slow wave) sleep.	1170	863	J21(RS4), D15(RS3), D03, D12
9. Paradoxical sleep.	1170	864	J10(RS2)
10. Sleep disorders.	1173	865	D98

CHAPTER 156: LIMBIC SYSTEM

Short Essays

1. Limbic system—components and functions.	1177	833	J15(RS3), J99, D06
2. Papez circuit.	1177	833	D19(RS3)
3. Motivation and addiction.	1181	834	J08(RS2)
4. List the features of 'Kluver-Bucy syndrome'.	1184	830	D13(RS3)

Short Answers

1. Limbic system—list the structures forming, their functions.	1177	833	J21(RS4), J00, D02, J03
2. Mention the effects of bilateral temporal lobectomy.	1184	830	J12
3. Describe Kluver-Bucy animal.	1184	830	D11, D14

CHAPTER 157: PHYSIOLOGY OF LEARNING AND MEMORY

Short Essays

1. Define learning. Explain the role of conditioned reflex in learning.	1186	869,873	D09, J14

Contd...

Contd...

	GKPAL	SEMBU	
2. Give classification of memory. Describe the mechanism of habituation.	1186	870	J10
3. What is conditioned reflex and unconditioned reflex? Explain with an example.	1187	873	D00, J03
4. Describe the molecular mechanisms of learning and memory.	1188	870,871	D16
Short Answers			
1. Types (classification) of memory with examples of each.	1186	870	J05
2. Habituation and sensitization.	1189	870, 871	J06(RS2)

CHAPTER 158: PHYSIOLOGY OF LANGUAGE AND SPEECH

Short Essays			
1. Name the language areas of cerebral cortex. Mention their location and explain their specific role. Give the features of lesion to these areas.	1194	875,877	J13, D13
2. Describe the mechanism of speech.	1194	875	D10
3. Discuss the role of Wernicke's area in production of speech.	1194	875	J09
4. How the speech of a person is affected with a lesion in 'Wernicke's area'.	1194	877	D17(RS3)
Short Answers			
1. Dyslexia.	—	—	J08(RS2)
2. Discuss the functions of angular gyrus.	1195	—	D10
3. Broca's area and mention its role in speech.	1195	876	D11(RS3), D98, J99
4. What is aphasia? What are the types? Name the center for speech.	1196	876	J11(RS2), J12(RS3), D01, J03, D04, D07, D11

CHAPTER 159: NEOCORTEX (ASSOCIATION CORTEX) AND CEREBRAL ASYMMETRY

Short Essay			
1. Concept of cerebral dominance (categorization of hemisphere).	1200	823	D07(RS2)

Contd...

PHYSIOLOGY

Contd...

	GKPAL	SEMBU	

CHAPTER 160: FUNCTIONS OF THE LOBES OF THE BRAIN AND CORTICAL PLASTICITY

Short Essays

	GKPAL	SEMBU	
1. Mention the various Brodman's (numbers) in the frontal lobe. Describe briefly each one.	1202	823	J06
2. Functions of prefrontal lobe.	1204	827	D10(RS2), D13(RS3)
3. What is frontal lobe syndrome and its behavioral effects?	1205	827	D11(RS3)

Short Answers

	GKPAL	SEMBU	
1. Functions of parietal lobe of the brain.	1203	827	D08(RS2)
2. Functions of prefrontal lobe.	1204	827	J04, D06, J10
3. Mention two effects of prefrontal lobotomy.	1205	827	D12

CHAPTER 161: CEREBROSPINAL FLUID

Long Essay

	GKPAL	SEMBU	
1. Describe the mechanism of secretion, circulation and functions of cerebrospinal fluid (CSF). Tabulate the composition of CSF against plasma. Discuss the clinical applications of CSF analysis.	1208, 1210	879	F21(RS4), D10(RS2), J10

Short Essay

	GKPAL	SEMBU	
1. Describe formation, circulation and function of cerebrospinal fluid (CSF). Add a note on hydrocephalus.	1208	879	J18(RS3), D15

Short Answers

	GKPAL	SEMBU	
1. Cerebrospinal fluid and its functions.	1207	879, 881	J09(RS2), J15(RS3), J02, J04, J05
2. Mention the site of production, drainage and method of collection of cerebrospinal fluid (CSF).	1208	879	J13
3. Lumbar puncture (sites and uses).	1210	881	J99, D03
4. Discuss papilledema.	1211	—	J08(RS2)
5. Explain blood-brain barrier in cerebral circulation.	1211	882	J09

Contd...

Contd...

	GKPAL	SEMBU	

SECTION 12: SPECIAL SENSES

PART A: VISION

CHAPTER 162: FUNCTIONAL ANATOMY OF EYE

Long Essay

1. Describe the formation, circulation, drainage and functions of aqueous humor. What is glaucoma?	1219	899,903	J03

Short Essays

1. Draw a diagram to show the different refractive media of the eye and explain their role in the dioptric power of the eye.	—	—	D05(RS2)
2. Describe the sources, circulation, drainage and functions of aqueous humor. Draw a diagram to show the circulation of aqueous humor. Give the significance of regulation of intraocular pressure.	1219	899,903	J05(RS2), D14(RS3), J17(RS3), D99, J04
3. Glaucoma—types.	1220	903	F21(RS4)
4. Importance of maintaining normal intraocular pressure.	1223	900	D17(RS3)

Short Answers

1. Describe the mechanism of constriction and dilation of pupil.	1219	897	J12
2. Name the intraocular muscles, with their functions.	1219	900	D99
3. Functions, circulation, absorption of aqueous humor and its applied aspect.	1219	899,903	J15(RS3), J99, J02, J08, J15, D15
4. Glaucoma.	1220	903	D12(RS3)
5. Mention the part of retina with highest visual acuity and give reasons for the same.	1222	899	J19(RS3)
6. What is fovea centralis and why it has highest visual acuity?	1222	899	D15, D16
7. Importance of fovea centralis.	1222	899	J15
8. Amacrine and horizontal cells.	1222	898	D09(RS2), J13(RS3)

Contd...

Contd...

	GKPAL	SEMBU	
9. What is the location and cause for physiological blind spot in visual field.	1222	898	D01, D04, J08
10. What is the normal intraocular pressure? What is the clinical importance?	1223	900,903	J11(RS2), D01, D02, D04
11. What is the normal intraocular pressure? How is it measured? Define glaucoma.	1223	900,903	D11(RS3)

CHAPTER 163: IMAGE-FORMING MECHANISM

Short Essays

1. Describe the errors of refraction and their correction.	1226	932	D07(RS2), D10(RS2), J11(RS2), J12(RS3), J14(RS3), D18(RS3), N20(RS3), D01, J08, D11
2. Draw diagram to show the formation of images in hypermetropia, myopia and astigmatism. Explain its correction.	1227	933	D06(RS2), D03

Short Answers

1. What are Purkinje Samson images? What do they demonstrate?	—	923	J00, J01
2. Accommodation in eye.	1225	922	J06(RS2)
3. Changes during accommodation for near vision (components of near response).	1226	924	J12(RS3), D05, D07
4. Define near point. Give its clinical significance.	1226	925	D14(RS3)
5. Myopia.	1227	933	D98
6. Hypermetropia—image formation and its correction (with help of a diaphragm).	1227	932	J09(RS2), D17(RS3), D10
7. Depict by means of sketches refractory errors in myopia and hypermetropia and their correction.	1227	932	D11(RS3), D13
8. What is astigmatism? Explain the basic defect in astigmatism. How is it corrected?	1227	934	J05

Contd...

Contd...

	GKPAL	SEMBU	
9. Presbyopia and its correction.	1227	934	J08(RS2), J99, J09, D12

CHAPTER 164: PHOTORECEPTOR MECHANISM

Short Essays

1. Distinguish between the functions of rods and cones. Explain how rhodopsin-retinene cycle.	—	906,908	D06
2. Scotopic vision.	—	907	D19(RS3)
3. Visual pigments.	1230	907	D12(RS3)
4. Describe the sequence of events in the photoreceptors when light strikes them.	1230	909	J12
5. Describe the sequence of events in phototransduction in rods and cones.	1230	909	D08
6. Describe the genesis of photoreceptor potential in rods.	1230	909	D14
7. Explain the ionic basis of photoreceptor potentials.	1230	909	D08

Short Answers

1. Differentiate rods from cones.	—	907	J16(RS3)
2. What is scotopic and photopic vision? What is Purkinje phenomenon?	—	907	D09, J14
3. Name the retinal receptors of vision (visual receptors). What are their functions?	1229	906	D13(RS3), J00, D00, J01, D07, D14
4. Name functions of rods and cones.	1229	907	D10(RS2)
5. Draw flowchart of rhodopsin—retinal visual cycle.	1232	908	D11

CHAPTER 165: VISUAL PATHWAY AND VISUAL CORTEX

Long Essay

1. Describe the optic pathway. What are the effects of lesions at various levels of the optic pathway?	1233	916, 918	J06

Contd...

PHYSIOLOGY

Contd...

	GKPAL	SEMBU	
Short Essays			
1. Describe visual pathway with a labeled diagram. Describe the effects of lesions at various levels in the pathway.	1233	916,918	J07(RS2), J10(RS2), D15(RS3), J18(RS3), J98, J10
2. Draw a labeled diagram of the visual pathway. Name the field defect produced by cutting the left optic tract and indicate it on a diagram.	1234	916, 920	D03
3. Draw the visual pathway. Explain homonymous hemianopia and macular sparing.	1234	916,920	J05(RS2)
4. Explain the disorders of visual field in relation to visual pathway.	1234	918	F21(RS4)
Short Answer			
1. Draw a visual pathway.	1234	918	J15(RS3)
Multiple Choice Questions			
1. Second order neuron in visual pathway is present in: a. Lateral geniculate body b. Pretectal area c. Optic nerve d. **Retina**	1235	916	J21(RS4)

CHAPTER 166: VISUAL ACUITY, VISUAL FIELD, LIGHT AND DARK ADAPTATIONS, AND VISUAL REFLEXES

Long Essay			
1. Describe the pupillary reflexes and their pathways. Add a note on Argyll-Robertson pupil.	1243, 1244	923,925	D15
Short Essays			
1. What is meant by visual acuity? What are the factors that influence visual acuity? Explain the physiological basis of testing visual acuity.	1240	912	D02, J08, D12
2. Name the different visual field defects caused by lesions to visual pathway. Give the basis of each defect. What is 'macular sparing'?	1241	918, 920	J13

Contd...

Contd...

	GKPAL	SEMBU	
3. Describe the mechanism of light and dark adaptation.	1242	910	D08
4. Dark adaptation—explain with help of a diagram, time course and changes occurring, factors contributing.	1242	910	D06(RS2), J10(RS2), J17(RS3), D00, J02, D04, J05, J09
5. What is homonymous hemianopia? Mention the lesions in the visual pathways that produce it.	1242	920,918	D10
6. Bitemporal hemianopia.	1242	919	D12(RS3)
7. Macular sparing.	1242	920	D09(RS2), J13(RS3)
8. What is the effect of lesion in visual pathway at the level of optic chiasma?	1242	919	J05
9. Dark adaptation and nyctalopia.	1242	910, 911	J16(RS3)
10. Light and accommodation reflexes (pupillary reflex).	1243	921,922	J09(RS2)
11. Explain pupillary light reflex. Describe the pathways involved in it.	1243	921	D10
12. Draw the pathway for 'light reflex' (direct/indirect).	1243	921	D13(RS3), J19(RS3)
13. Draw a diagram to show the pathways for light reflexes (no explanation needed).	1243	921	D06(RS2), D05
14. Accommodation reflex—trace the pathway and explain the changes occurring during accommodation. What is Argyll-Robertsons pupil?	1243	924	D09(RS2), J13(RS3), J17(RS3), J01, J07
15. Describe the mechanism of accommodation. Draw and label accommodation pathway (near response).	1243, 1244	924	J15(RS3), J04
Short Answers			
1. Define: (i) Visual acuity; (ii) Accommodation.	1240, 1243	912,924	D99
2. Visual acuity—define, basis, expression.	1240	912	D19(RS3), J01, J05, D05
3. What is field of vision? What are the limits of field of vision in different meridians?	1241	913	J02
4. Describe the dark and light adaptation.	1242	910	D11

Contd...

Contd...

	GKPAL	SEMBU	
5. Dark adaptation—physiological basis, three mechanism involved, dark adaption curve, related disorder.	1242	910	J14(RS3), J98, J13
6. What is nyctalopia? Give its physiological basis.	1243	911	D13
7. Accommodation reflex (near response of eye).	1243	924	J07(RS2), D98, J99, D09, J14, J15
8. What is Argyl-Robertson's pupil? Name site of lesion producing it.	1244	925	D00, D02

CHAPTER 167: COLOR VISION

Long Essay

1. What are the mechanisms to perceive color vision (theories of color vision)? Add a note on color blindness (classification and tests).	1245	927	J06(RS2)

Short Essays

1. Color vision.	1245	927	J98
2. Theories of color vision (mechanisms of color vision).	1245	928	D08(RS2), D16
3. Describe the Young-Helmoltz theory of color vision.	1246	928	D10
4. Describe color blindness.	1247	930	J12(RS3), D15(RS3), N20(RS3)
5. Define and classify color blindness. What is the peculiarity of inheritance of color blindness?	1247	930	J00, J02, D04

Short Answers

1. Explain primary and complementary colors.	1245	928	J10
2. Explain briefly trichromatic theory of color vision?	1246	928	D99, J06
3. Color blindness.	1247	930	D06

CHAPTER 168: MOVEMENTS OF THE EYE

Short Answers

1. Strabismus.	—	—	J07

Contd...

Contd...

	GKPAL	SEMBU	
2. Describe the innervation and movements of extraocular muscles.	1250	901	D08
3. Mechanism of depth perception of object by the eyes.	1252	—	J08(RS2)

CHAPTER 169: ELECTRO-OCULOGRAPHY, ELECTRORETINOGRAPHY AND VISUAL-EVOKED POTENTIALS

None

PART B: HEARING

CHAPTER 170: FUNCTIONAL ANATOMY AND FUNCTIONS OF THE EAR

Short Essays

1. Attenuation reflex.	—	937	J07
2. Describe the structure, contents and functions of middle ear. Explain the tympanic reflex (impedance matching).	1256	936,937	J21(RS4), D09(RS2),, J11(RS2), J12(RS3), J13(RS3), D15(RS3), J16(RS3), D17(RS3), J00, D06, J12, D16
3. Describe the functions of tympanic membrane and middle ear ossicles.	1257	936	J08(RS2), D05
4. Describe briefly the functions of middle ear.	1258	936	J10(RS2), J18(RS3), D18(RS3), D98, D99, D12
5. Explain 'impedance matching' and give its significance.	1258	937,944	D06(RS2), J09(RS2), J99, D11
6. Explain the functions of organ of Corti—labeled diagram, functions.	1259	939	D11(RS3), J13
7. Describe the structure of organ of Corti and explain the functioning of/ mechanism of stimulation of hair cells.	1259	939	J98, J09, J15

Contd...

PHYSIOLOGY

Contd...

	GKPAL	SEMBU	
Short Answers			
1. Differentiate endolymph from perilymph.	—	939	J16(RS3)
2. Write briefly the structures in the middle ear. How it is connected to nasopharynx and what is its importance?	1256	936	D07
3. Name the ear ossicles. Mention their role in hearing (sound transmission).	1257	936	J13, D15
4. Describe the functions of middle ear ossicles.	1257	936	J09
5. Functions of middle ear.	1258	936	J10, D11
6. Attenuation reflex (tympanic reflex) and its importance.	1258	937	D11(RS3), D19(RS3), N20(RS3), J98, J03, J05, J08, D10
7. Attenuation reflex and impedance matching.	1258	937, 944	D11(RS3), D19(RS3), N20(RS3), J98, J03, J05, J08, D10
8. Describe impedance matching.	1258	944	J12(RS3), J14(RS3), J19(RS3), D00, J01, J02, D06
9. Draw and label the transverse section of cochlea.	1259	938	J15
10. Describe organ of Corti with a labeled diagram.	1259	939	D15(RS3), D18(RS3), D99, J06, D09, J14

CHAPTER 171: AUDITORY PATHWAYS

Short Essay			
1. Describe auditory pathway (pathway of hearing) with a labeled diagram and list two special features of this pathway.	1262	941	J05(RS2), J99, D00, D01, J02, D04, J06, J08

Contd...

Contd...

	GKPAL	SEMBU	
Short Answers			
1. Presbycusis.	—	942	D16(RS3)
2. Name auditory cortical area.	1263	942	D00
Multiple Choice Questions			
1. The primary auditory cortex is situated in: a. Frontal lobe b. Parietal lobe c. **Temporal lobe** d. Occipital lobe	1263	942	J21(RS4)

CHAPTER 172: MECHANISM OF HEARING

Short Essays			
1. Explain pitch (different intensities of sound) discrimination by the human ear (role of 'cochlea').	1265	946	D05(RS2), D13(RS3), J19(RS3), D03
2. Describe the role of inner ear in the mechanism of hearing.	1266	944	J10
3. Endocochleal/endolymphatic potential—genesis, factors affecting.	1269	946	J07, D09, J14
Short Answers			
1. Masking.	1266	—	J06(RS2)
2. What is endocochlear potential?	1267	946	J17(RS3)
3. Explain the mechanism of localization of sound.	1269	947	J12

CHAPTER 173: HEARING DEFECTS AND HEARING TESTS

Short Essays			
1. Describe a normal audiogram.	—	949	D05(RS2)
2. Explain how audiometry is superior to Tuning forks test.	—	949	J04
3. What is meant by deafness? What are the different types of deafness and its causes? How is it tested?	1271	948	D02
4. Sensorineural deafness.	1271	948	D14(RS3)
5. Hearing tests and their physiological basis.	1272	948	D07(RS2), J09(RS2), J05

Contd...

PHYSIOLOGY

Contd...

	GKPAL	SEMBU	
6. Three tuning fork tests of hearing.	1272	949	J07(RS2)
Short Answers			
1. How is 'conduction deafness' differentiated from 'nerve deafness'.	—	948	D13
2. Explain the differences between conduction deafness and sensorineural deafness.	—	948	D05
3. Draw an audiogram of a normal individual and compare it with that of a person with 'conduction deafness'.	—	949	D13(RS3)
4. What are types of deafness? Give an example for each.	1271	948	D14
5. Conduction deafness.	1271	948	D98
6. Mention the (utility of) tuning fork tests used to assess deafness	1272	949	F21(RS4), J21(RS4)
7. Rinne's test and its interpretation.	1272	949	D07(RS2), J01
8. Explain Weber's test and its application.	1272	949	D00, D01, D04, D10
9. What is meant by audiometry?	1272	949	J03, J12, D12

PART C: SMELL AND TASTE

CHAPTER 174: PHYSIOLOGY OF SMELL

Short Essays			
1. Primary sensation of smell.	—	—	J07
2. Neural pathway and the physiological role of olfaction.	1276	955	D13(RS3)
3. Describe with the help of a diagram, the olfactory pathway (pathway for smell). Explain the term adaptation in relation to olfaction.	1276	955	J09(RS2), D19(RS3), D02, D03, J12
Short Answers			
1. Name any two special features of olfactory sensation.	1275	954	D15
2. Mention the location of olfactory receptors. What is olfactory adaptation?	1275	954	J13

Contd...

Contd...

	GKPAL	SEMBU	
3. Draw and label olfactory receptor cell.	1276	955	N20(RS3)
4. Olfactory bulb.	1276	955	J98
5. Draw and label basic neural circuits in olfactory bulb.	1276	955	D08
6. Name the cortical olfactory areas.	1276	955	D14(RS3)
7. Draw and label olfactory pathway.	1277	955	J11(RS2), J14(RS3), J15
8. List the factors affecting olfaction.	1278	—	D16
9. What are anosmia and hyposmia? Mention any common cause.	1278	956	D15

CHAPTER 175: PHYSIOLOGY OF TASTE

Short Essays

1. Describe the structure of taste bud, the location of taste buds and the taste pathway.	1280	950	D11(RS3)
2. Describe the taste pathways and mechanism of taste perception (physiological role).	1281	951	D12(RS3), J15(RS3), J19(RS3), J00, D00, J03, D06, J09, D11, D14
3. Taste pathway and taste disorders.	1281	951	D18(RS3)
4. Name the primary taste sensations. Give the role of chemical senses in humans.	1281	952	J04
5. Draw a diagram to show the taste pathway from the anterior two-thirds of the tongue.	1282	951	D05(RS2)
6. Mention the basic modalities of taste sensation and their representation on the tongue. Describe a taste bud.	1281	952	D01

Short Answers

1. Taste buds.	1280	950	J10(RS2), J18(RS3), J99
2. Draw neat labeled diagram of taste receptor.	1281	951	J21(RS4)
3. Mention the nerve supply of the tongue which carries the general sensations and taste sensations from different areas of the tongue.	1282	951	D02

Contd...

PHYSIOLOGY

Contd...

	GKPAL	SEMBU	
4. Name basic taste sensations. On what part of the tongue they are perceived?	1281	952	J10
5. Name the primary taste sensation. Explain the mechanism of perception of any one taste sensation.	1281	952	D17(RS3)
6. Name the primary taste sensations. What is ageusia?	1281	952, 953	J11(RS2), D14(RS3), D12
7. Draw taste pathway from anterior two-thirds of tongue to the cortex.	1282	951	J16(RS3)
8. Draw a labeled diagram of pathways for taste.	1282	951	D10(RS2), D15(RS3), N20(RS3), D99, J02, J03, D10
9. What is ageusia? Trace the pathway of taste up to the taste center.	1284	953,951	D07

SECTION 13: INTEGRATIVE PHYSIOLOGY

CHAPTER 176: STRUCTURE AND FUNCTIONS OF THE SKIN

Short Essay

1. Explain briefly the role of skin in regulation of body temperature.	1291	330	D10(RS2), J15

Short Answers

1. Draw and label the structure of skin.	1289	326	J07
2. Sweat gland.	1290	328	J09(RS2), D10(RS2)
3. Name the different types of sweat glands and give the stimulus for each.	1290	328	D03
4. Eccrine sweat glands—distribution and functions.	1290	328	D17(RS3), D08
5. Functions of skin.	1291	329	J12(RS3), D14(RS3), D98, D99, D02, J03, D06, D09, J11, J13, D13, J14, D14
6. What are the secretory and synthetic functions of skin?	1291	330	D11(RS3)

Contd...

Contd...

	GKPAL	SEMBU	
7. Describe the functions of skin in regulation of body temperature.	1291	330	D11

CHAPTER 177: REGULATION OF BODY TEMPERATURE AND ACCLIMATIZATION TO HOT AND COLD ENVIRONMENTS

Short Essays

	GKPAL	SEMBU	
1. Role of conduction type of heat loss in treating heat stroke.	—	333	J08(RS2)
2. How much is normal body temperature and explain the various heat gain mechanisms.	1294, 1296	331,332	J11
3. What is core and shell temperature? Explain heat loss mechanisms.	1294, 1297	331,333	J15(RS3)
4. Explain the heat loss mechanisms to maintain constant body temperature.	1297	332	J07(RS2), D07
5. Regulation of body temperature.	1298	332	J18(RS3)
6. Mechanisms activated in body with exposure to heat. What is heat stroke?	1301	333	J14(RS3)
7. Immediate cardiovascular changes on exposure to hot climate.	1301	333	D07(RS2)
8. How is body temperature defended when a person is exposed to very cold environment?	1301	332	J15
9. Body mechanisms activated with exposure to cold.	1301	332	J16(RS3)
10. Cardiovascular changes on exposure to cold.	1303	332	D08(RS2)
11. List the beneficial effects of fever.	1304	335	F21(RS4)
12. Hypothermia.	1305	335	J98, J99
13. What is hypothermia and what is the clinical importance of induced hypothermia?	1305	335	D07

Short Answers

	GKPAL	SEMBU	
1. Role of horripilation.	—	—	D03
2. Core and shell temperature.	1294	331	D10
3. What is normal body temperature? What is the role of skin in maintaining it.	1294, 1291	331	J01
4. Explain the factors affecting body temperature.	1294	331	J08

Contd...

Contd...

	GKPAL	SEMBU	
5. What is the normal body temperature? Enumerate the bodily reactions that tend to prevent a rise in body temperature.	1294, 1296	331	J02
6. What is the normal "core body temperature"? Mention the ways in which the body can gain heat.	1294, 1296	331	D01, D04
7. What is the normal body temperature? What are the means of heat loss from the body?	1294, 1297	331	D02
8. Physiological mechanisms of heat gain (modes of heat production).	1296	332	J19(RS3), D99
9. Explain the heat loss mechanisms.	1297	333	D13(RS3), J17(RS3), J00, J03, J08
10. Explain how sweating helps in temperature regulation.	1297	333	D05(RS2), J04, D06
11. How does sweating help in regulating body temperature? Give the innervation of eccrine sweat glands.	1297	333	D12
12. Explain how behavioral thermoregulation operates to maintain body temperature.	1298	—	J09
13. Name the hypothalamic centers that regulate body temperature. Mention the role of hypothalamus in the causing fever.	1299	333	J13
14. Explain the mechanism of temperature regulation by anterior hypothalamus.	1299	797	D10
15. Explain the role of hypothalamus in thermoregulation in cold environment.	1299	797	J12
16. What is the role of epinephrine on thermogenesis?	1295	—	D16
17. What are the physiologic thermoregulatory mechanisms activated by an increase in body temperature or exposure to heat?	1297	333	D01, D04, J05, D08
18. Brown fat—functions.	1301	332	J07(RS2), D15
19. Enumerate the thermoregulatory changes when a person is exposed to 20 degree centigrade.	1301	333	D13
20. How is body temperature defended when a person is exposed to very cold environment?	1301	333	D05, J10, D14

Contd...

Contd...

	GKPAL	SEMBU	
21. Explain the role of shivering in temperature regulation.	1301	332	J05(RS2)
22. Nonshivering thermogenesis.	1301	—	D12(RS3)
23. What is pyrexia? Explain the physiological basis of its genesis.	1303	335	J12
24. Describe pathogenesis and functions of fever.	1303	335	J10, D12
25. Endogenous pyrogens.	1303	335	D09(RS2), J13(RS3)
26. What is malignant hyperthermia.	1305	—	N20(RS3)
27. Heat stroke—explain (symptoms and treatment).	1305	—	J09, D09, J14
28. Describe the effects and use of hypothermia.	1305	335	D11

CHAPTER 178: AVIATION AND SPACE PHYSIOLOGY

Short Answer

1. Positive 'G'	1308	—	D08(RS2)

CHAPTER 179: PHYSIOLOGY OF EXERCISE AND SPORTS SCIENCE

Long Essay

1. Describe the cardiorespiratory adaptations to exercise.	1320, 1317	616, 693	D09

Short Essays

1. Explain the cardiorespiratory changes during exercise.	1320, 1317	616,693	J21(RS4), J06, J10
2. Explain the changes which occur in the respiratory system during muscular exercise.	1317	693	J05(RS2)
3. Describe the oxygen debt mechanism.	1317	694	D08
4. Describe the cardiovascular changes during muscular exercise.	1320	616	J12(RS3)
5. Describe the circulatory changes during muscular exercise.	1320	616	J00, J01, D01, J04
6. Describe the effect of muscular exercise on coronary blood flow.	1321	616	D05
7. Describe physiological effects of physical training.	1323	614, 693	F21(RS4)

Contd...

Contd...

	GKPAL	SEMBU	
Short Answers			
1. Oxygen debt.	1317	694	J06
2. Diagrammatically represent the ventilatory changes during exercise.	1317	693	J09(RS2)
3. Describe the effects of dynamic exercise on muscle blood flow.	1321	616	J07
4. Why do heart rate and rate of respiration increase during exercise?	1320, 1317	616, 693	J09

CHAPTER 180: PRINCIPLES OF ACID-BASE HOMEOSTASIS

Short Essays			
1. Renal regulation of H^+ ion.	1328	301	J10(RS2)
2. Outline the role of kidneys in acid-base balance. Add a note on tubular buffers.	1328,763	302	D12, D13
3. Enumerate the causes of metabolic acidosis. How is it corrected?	1329	304	D07
4. Renal compensation in respiratory acidosis.	1329	304	D05(RS2)
Short Answers			
1. What is the pH value of arterial and venous blood? Name one physiological and one abnormal condition producing alkalosis.	1326	304	J07
2. Bicarbonate buffer system.	1327	302	D08(RS2)
3. Metabolic acidosis.	1329	304	J08(RS2)

CHAPTER 181: PHYSIOLOGY OF GROWTH AND DEVELOPMENT

Long Essays			
1. Give a detailed account of physiology of growth and development in human beings.	1332	349	J98
2. Describe in detail endocrine regulation of growth.	1333	349	J04
Short Essay			
1. Describe the mechanism by which hormones regulate growth.	1333	349	D06

Contd...

Contd...

	GKPAL	SEMBU	
Short Answer			
1. What is Lorain Dwarfism and its causes?	1335	349	D15

CHAPTER 182: PRINCIPLES OF ENERGY METABOLISM

None.

CHAPTER 183: PHYSIOLOGY OF NUTRITION

Short Essay			
1. Dietary fiber.	—	262	J09(RS2)
Short Answers			
1. What is respiratory quotient and the effect of metabolism of various food stuffs on its value?	—	—	D11(RS3)
2. What is dietary fiber? What is its importance?	—	260	D18(RS3), J19(RS3), D08, D09
3. Vitamin K.	1341	120	D08(RS2)
4. Why is blood clotting abnormal in patients with vitamin K deficiency?	1341	120	D07(RS2)
5. What is the effect of vitamin K deficiency on coagulation?	1341	120	D15

CHAPTER 184: PHYSIOLOGY OF AGING AND OXIDATIVE STRESS

None

CHAPTER 185: PHYSIOLOGY OF YOGA AND PREVENTION OF AGING

None

CHAPTER 186: MISCELLANEOUS

Long Essay			
1. Discuss the hypothalamo-hypophyseal control of ovulation and spermatogenesis.	—	—	D06
Short Essays			
1. Define 'pitting edema'. Give its physiological basis.	66	—	J13

Contd...

PHYSIOLOGY

Contd...

	GKPAL	SEMBU	
2. Problems in prematurity.	—	—	J08(RS2)
3. Smell and taste are linked—explain.	—	—	D09(RS2), J13(RS3)
4. Reactive hyperemia.	461	585	J10(RS2)
5. Explain the role of 'chemical senses' in humans.		—	J05(RS2)
Short Answers			
1. Define lifestyle disorders. Mention the health effects of sedentary lifestyle.	—	—	J21(RS4)
2. AS Paintal.	558	—	J06
3. Factors causing hypoeffective heart.	—	—	D08(RS2)
4. What is translocation blood and when is it taking place in a normal subject?	—	—	J09
5. Physiological basis of use of a drug in the treatment of stroke.	—	—	D08(RS2)
6. Enumerate the types of RNA and explain their functions.	35	—	J11
7. What is meant by translation and transcription process?	34	—	D01, J03, D04
8. What are the causes for latent period in simple muscle twitch?	262	—	D15
9. Enumerate the functions of medulla oblongata.	1126	—	J08
10. Name some abnormal involuntary movements and the sites of lesion.	1137	—	D15
11. Carbon monoxide poisoning.	551	—	J13(RS3)
12. What is transferrin?	702	75	J15
13. What is reactive hyperemia? Where does it occur?	461	585	D10
14. Superfemale.	944	—	J19(RS3)
15. In which conditions tremors are observed and how they are differentiated?	1138	790, 818, 844	D11(RS3)
16. Name any two types of abnormal gaits. Mention the diseases associated with them.	1138, 1146	382, 765, 818	D02

3

BIOCHEMISTRY

REFERENCES

1. U Satyanaran, U Chakrapani **(STNRN)**: Biochemistry (6th Edition), Elsevier Health Sciences, New Delhi, ₹ 1825/-
2. DM Vasudevan, Sreekumari S, Kannan Vaidyanathan **(VSDN)**: Textbook of Biochemistry (For Medical Students), (10th Edition Revised Reprint), Jaypee Brothers Medical Publishers (P) Ltd, New Delhi, ₹ 1750/-

Curriculum

STNRN VSDN

SECTION 1: CHEMICAL CONSTITUENT OF LIFE

CHAPTER 1: BIOMOLECULES AND THE CELL

Short Essays

1. Draw a neat labeled diagram of a cell with the subcellular organelles. Explain the functions of each (any four organelles).	5	13	J21(RS4), D12(RS3), J19(RS3)
2. Mitochondrial structure and important functions.	6	16	D05
3. Lysosomes.	7	15	J07

Short Answers

1. Mitochondria.	6	16	J12(RS3)
2. Endoplasmic reticulum.	6	14	J10(RS2)
3. Give metabolic function of endoplasmic reticulum and mitochondria.	6	16	J07(RS2)
4. Lysosomes (metabolic functions, markers and clinical significance).	7	15	D10(RS2), D19(RS3), D16
5. Name subcellular organelles. Which are metabolic functions of cytosols?	8	16	J05(RS2)

Multiple Choice Questions

1. Which of the following subcellular organelle is involved in protein sorting? a. Lysosome b. **Golgi apparatus** c. Peroxisomes d. Ribosomes	7	14	J21(RS4)

CHAPTER 2: CARBOHYDRATES

Short Essays

1. Function of carbohydrates.	9	90	D08(RS2)
2. Classify carbohydrates with two examples for each class and subclass.	9	90	J19(RS3)
3. Monosaccharides.	10	92	D19(RS3)
4. Epimerization.	12	92	J11
5. Invert sugar.	19	96	J98
6. Polysaccharides.	20	97	J00
7. Describe the structure and biomedical importance of homopolysaccharides.	21	97	J02

Contd...

BIOCHEMISTRY

Contd...

	STNRN	VSDN	
8. What are mucopolysaccharides (glycosaminoglycans)? Give their biomedical importance with examples (name the functions and composition of four mucopolysaccharides).	23	98	D15(RS3), J16(RS3), J04, J12
9. What are mucopolysaccharides? a. Name the mucopolysaccharide present in the glomerular basement membrane. What is its significance? b. Explain the biochemical basis of heparin as anticoagulant. c. Write the composition and importance of chondroitin sulfate. d. Which mucopolysaccharide maintains the transparency of cornea?	23	98	F21(RS4)
10. Chondroitin sulfate.	25	99	J99, D04
Short Answers			
1. Benedict's test and its importance.	—	93	J12
2. Compare and contrast starch and glycogen.	—	—	D15(RS3), J00
3. Epimerism and anomerism.	12	92	J14(RS3)
4. What are epimers? Give examples (name two epimers of alpha D-glucose).	12	92	D07
5. Mutarotation.	14	92	D06(RS2), J06
6. Detection of reducing sugar in urine.	16	93	J02
7. Glycosidic linkage.	18	—	J09
8. What is the clinical importance of glycosides?	18	94	D06
9. Invert sugar.	19	96	D14, D15
10. Milk sugar.	20	96	D00
11. Mention four homopolysaccharides.	21	97	D09
12. Amylose and amylopectins.	21	97	D00
13. Animal homopolysaccharide.	22	98	J98
14. Glycosaminoglycans.	23	98	J06(RS2), J08, J14
15. Heteropolysaccharides.	23	98	D98, D11
16. Give the composition of hyaluronic acid.	24	98	J13
17. Name mucopolysaccharides. Mention their functions.	25	98	J05(RS2)
18. Write the composition of any two heteropolysaccharides.	25	98	D12

Contd...

Contd...

	STNRN	VSDN	
19. Name the mucopolysaccharide with anticoagulant activity. Write its composition and its mechanism of action.	25	98	J21(RS4)
Multiple Choice Questions			
1. All are an example of monosaccharide, *except:* a. Glucose b. Galactose c. **Trehalose** d. Mannose	11	92	J21(RS4)
CHAPTER 3: LIPIDS			
Long Essay			
1. Define lipids. Classify lipids with an example for each. Mention the functions of the lipids.	29	104	D12(RS3)
Short Essays			
1. Classify of lipid with examples. What are essential fatty acids? Mention one function of each.	108	104, 106	D11
2. Compound lipids.	29	108	D98
3. What are essential fatty acids? what are the functions of essential fatty acids?	32	106	D16(RS3)
4. Phospholipids—define, classify with examples, significance (functions), composition and functions of any two.	35	108	D09(RS2), D01, D03, J04, J08, D10, J12
Short Answers			
1. Unsaturated fatty acid (two examples).	30	106	D05, J09
2. Essential fatty acids and their importance.	32	106	D05(RS2), D15(RS3), J99, J00, D07, D08, D12, J14, J15
3. Triglycerides.	33	107	J98
4. Rancidity.	34	108	J08(RS2), J06
5. Lipid peroxidation—clinical importance.	34	223	D07(RS2)
6. Phospholipids (name any two with their composition and functions).	35	108	D13(RS3), D06, J10, D12
7. Lecithin.	37	110	J99
8. Sphingolipids.	37	112	D19(RS3)
9. Name the components of sphingomyelin.	37	112	D13
10. What are the components of ceramide? Name a phospholipid which contains ceramide.	37	112	J07

Contd...

Contd...

	STNRN	VSDN	
11. Surfactant—composition and function.	38	110	J02, J15
12. Deficiency of lung surfactant causes respiratory distress syndrome. a. What is the composition of lung surfactant? b. What is the biochemical basis for respiratory distress syndrome? c. What is the significance of L/S ratio.	38	110	F21(RS4)
13. Gangliosides.	38	112	J98
Multiple Choice Questions			
1. ___________ is the nitrogen containing phospholipid. a. **Phosphatidylcholine** b. Phosphatidylinositol c. Phosphatidylglycerol d. Diphosphatidylglycerol	37	110	J21(RS4)
CHAPTER 4: PROTEINS AND AMINO ACIDS			
Long Essay			
1. Classify amino acid based on their structure giving examples.	46	30	J14(RS3)
Short Essays			
1. Classify amino acids based on their nutritional significance giving examples. What are non protein amino acids? Give one example.	50	32	J21(RS4)
2. Essential amino acids.	50	32	D09(RS2)
3. Describe the decarboxylation reactions of amino acids with four examples. Give its significance.	53	35	J11(RS2), J17(RS3)
4. Structural organization of proteins.	55	37	J09, D12
5. Explain the structure and function relationship of protein with an example.	55	41	F21(RS4)
6. Define primary, secondary, tertiary and quaternary structure of protein. What are the noncovalent forces which preserve the secondary structure?	55	37	D11(RS3)
7. Secondary structure of proteins.	59	38	J08(RS2), J07
8. Give the salient features of α-helical structure and quaternary structure of proteins.	59	39	D13

Contd...

Contd...

	STNRN	VSDN	
9. Describe the bonds that contribute to (stabilize) protein structure.	61	37	J98, D03
10. Classify proteins based on their function giving an example for each class.	67	45	J13(RS3)
11. Biologically active peptides (biological importance of peptides).	68	46	J08, D16
12. Glutathione.	68	46	D99
Short Answers			
1. Name two hydroxy amino acids.	49	30	J07
2. Nutritional classification of amino acids.	50	32	J10(RS2)
3. Essential amino acids and their importance (functions).	50	32	J11(RS2), D98, J09, J03, J06, D09, D10,
4. Mention two/four nonprotein amino acids and their significance.	54	31	D03, J08
5. Peptide bond.	56	37	J10
6. Secondary structure of proteins.	59	38	D13(RS3), D10
7. Tertiary and quaternary structure of proteins.	61	39	D14(RS3)
8. Give brief account on quaternary structure of proteins.	61	41	J05(RS2)
9. Bonds stabilizing protein structure.	61	37	J15(RS3)
10. What is isoelectric pH? What is the application of isoelectric pH? State properties of a protein at its isoelectric pH.	64	33, 44	D19(RS3), J07, D07, J13
11. Name two agents used to precipitate proteins.	64	44	J07
12. What is biuret reaction? What is its application?	65	46	J99, D01
13. Denaturation of proteins and factors causing denaturation.	65	44	J10(RS2), J15(RS3), D16(RS3), J99, J08, J11, D12
14. What is heat coagulation test? What is its clinical application?	66	44	J03
15. Functional classification of proteins.	67	45	D07(RS2)
16. What is complete protein?	68	46	D09(RS2)
17. Biologically active peptides and their functions.	68	46	J06(RS2), D06
18. Glutathione and its significance (role in erythrocytes).	68	46	D12(RS3), D16(RS3), D12

Contd...

Contd...

	STNRN	VSDN	
Multiple Choice Questions			
1. The protein part present in nucleoprotein is: a. Globin b. Opsin c. **Histones** d. Apoferritin	—	46	J21(RS4)
CHAPTER 5: NUCLEIC ACIDS AND NUCLEOTIDES			
Long Essay			
1. Draw neat diagram of Watson Crick model of DNA, explain its characteristics and the bonds that play a role in the stability of DNA structure.	77	636	J15(RS3)
Short Essays			
1. Structure and function of DNA.	76	635	D01, J08
2. RNA—types, salient features and functions.	81	651	J13(RS3)
3. Structure and functions of mRNA.	81	652	J11(RS2)
4. Name the RNA which carries amino acids to the site of protein biosynthesis. With illustration explain the structure.	83	657	J21(RS4)
5. Structure and functions of tRNA. Mention the unusual bases present in it.	83	657	D13(RS3), J18(RS3), J01, D06, D12
Short Answers			
1. Compare and contrast between nucleosides and nucleotides.	—	—	F21(RS4)
2. Distinguish between RNA and DNA.	—	637	D05(RS2), D19(RS3), J06, J12
3. Cyclic nucleotides.	—	620	J06(RS2), J11
4. Mention the functions of DNA.	72	636	J02
5. Which are biologically important nucleotides? Mention their functions.	73	—	J05(RS2), D05
6. Name four adenosine derivatives.	75	—	D01
7. Salient features of Chargaff's rule.	77	636	D10, D15
8. Salient features of Watson-Crick model of DNA.	77	636	D11

Contd...

Contd...

	STNRN	VSDN	
9. Base pairing rule and Wobble hypothesis.	78	636	J13(RS3)
10. Base pairing rule and its importance.	78	636	D07(RS2), J14
11. Different types of RNA with their function.	81	651	J19(RS3)
12. Messenger RNA (mRNA)—structure and functions.	81	652	J98, J05, J08
13. Ribosomal RNA.	83	658	J15(RS3)
14. Structure of tRNA.	83	657	N20(RS3)
15. Draw a neat labeled diagram of tRNA.	83	657	F21(RS4), D14(RS3
16. Types of RNA and their function.	84	652	J07(RS2), D00, J09
17. What is the role of tRNA?	84	657	D09

CHAPTER 6: ENZYMES

Long Essays

1. What are enzymes? Classify enzymes with one example each. Explain any four factors that affect enzyme activity. Add a note on enzyme specificity.	87, 90, 98	56, 65, 73	J13(RS3), J14
2. Classify enzymes giving an example with the reaction catalyzed.	88	57	D15(RS3)
3. Explain the influence of various factors on enzyme activity.	90	65	D06(RS2), D16(RS3)
4. Define the enzyme inhibition. Explain the features of competitive and non -competitive inhibition. Mention the therapeutic importance of competitive inhibition.	94	68	D16
5. Define isoenzymes. Mention the principles used for separation of isoenzymes. Write about the clinical importance of isoenzymes.	112	75	D07(RS2)

Short Essays

1. Define and classify enzymes (IUB classification) with one example for each class indicating the reaction catalyzed.	88	57	J21(RS4), J18(RS3), J02, D09, J11, J12
2. Factors affecting enzyme action (reaction).	90	65	D06, D10

Contd...

BIOCHEMISTRY

Contd...

	STNRN	VSDN	
3. K_m value (Michaelis-Menten constant) of an enzyme and its significance with a suitable example.	90	66	D10(RS2), J12(RS3), J08
4. Explain the effect of temperature and substrate concentration on enzyme activity with a graph.	90	66	F21(RS4)
5. Temperature and pH as factors affecting velocity of enzyme catalyzed reactions, with examples.	91	68	J19(RS3), J10
6. Describe the various type of enzyme inhibition giving suitable examples.	94	68	D18(RS3)
7. Explain competitive and noncompetitive inhibition with examples. Mention significance of competitive inhibition.	94	68	J07(RS2), N20(RS3)
8. Competitive inhibition—features, examples, importance in medicine (clinical use).	94	68	D08(RS2), J99, D02, D04, D07, D14
9. Noncompetitive enzyme inhibition.	96	68	J10(RS2)
10. Explain enzyme specificities with examples.	98	73	J12(RS3), J15
11. Coenzyme and their role in metabolism with four examples.	99	58	J07, J09
12. Describe the regulation of enzyme activity.	103	68	J04, J05
13. Allosteric enzymes.	103	71	J14(RS3), D99
14. Explain the mechanism of action of allosteric enzymes? Name the allosteric inhibitor and allosteric activator for phosphofructokinase and acetyl CoA—carboxylase.	103	71	D11(RS3)
15. Proenzymes.	105	68	D98
16. Therapeutic uses of enzymes.	108	80	J05(RS2)
17. Diagnostic importance of enzymes (enzymes in clinical diagnosis)—diagnostic enzymology.	110	80	J11(RS2), J08, D08, D12, D13
18. How does estimation of enzymes in serum help in clinical diagnosis (clinical significance of serum enzyme estimation)? Illustrate with five examples.	110	80	J01
19. Name five enzymes of diagnostic significance. Give the normal serum level and one clinical condition associated with their increase.	110	80	D01

Contd...

BIOCHEMISTRY

Contd...

	STNRN	VSDN	
20. Isoenzymes and their clinical importance citing three examples.	112	75	D05(RS2), J16(RS3), J17(RS3), D17(RS3), D16
21. What are isoenzymes? Discuss the isoenzyme forms of LDH.	112	75	D15
22. What are isoenzymes? Name the isoenzymes forms of LDH and CK. What is their clinical significance?	112	75	J03
23. What are isoenzymes? Write the isoenzymes of CPK with tissue distribution. Which isoenzyme is cardiac specific and write its pattern of rise in patients with myocardial infarction.	112, 115	75, 262	F21(RS4)
24. What are isoenzymes? Explain the enzyme profile in myocardial infarction.	112, 115	75, 262	D11
25. Clinical importance of enzymes in assessment of cardiac disease and liver function.	115	76, 262	D13(RS3)
26. Name three enzymes commonly estimated in myocardial infarction. Give its importance and limitations.	115	262	D14(RS3)
27. Diagnostic enzymes used in the assessment of different liver functions.	115	76	D15(RS3)
Short Answers			
1. Classify enzymes with suitable examples.	88	57	J01, D04, J06
2. Lyases.	89	58	J98
3. K_m value of enzymes and its significance.	90	66	D05(RS2), J01, D04, D08, J11, J13
4. Explain the relationship between K_m and affinity.	91	66	D16(RS3)
5. Explain how change in temp alters the enzyme activity.	91	67	J00
6. Explain how change in pH alters the enzyme activity.	92	67	D00
7. Competitive inhibition of enzyme activity (give two examples).	94	67	J16(RS3), D05

Contd...

Contd...

	STNRN	VSDN	
8. Methanol poisoning can be alleviated by ethanol, justify.	94	—	J06(RS2)
9. Mention the actions and uses of two competitive enzyme inhibitors.	95	68	J03, D03
10. Define absolute specificity of enzyme. Give two examples.	98	73	D02
11. Coenzymes (mention three with their functions).	99	58	D13(RS3), D19(RS3)
12. What is meant by lock and key mechanism of enzymes?	101	61	D09
13. Define allosteric enzyme with an example and name modulators for the enzyme.	103	71	D06, D12
14. Define zymogens (proenzymes). Give two examples.	105	67	D09(RS2), J00, D02, J03, J04, D08, D10
15. What are ribozymes? Mention one use of ribozymes.	108	656	D09
16. Give three/two examples of enzymes having therapeutic use and indicate their specific applications.	108	80	D12(RS3), D02
17. Enzymes of diagnostic importance.	110	80	J13(RS3), J09, D14
18. Serum amylase and its diagnostic significance.	111	77	J10(RS2), J99
19. Mention the significance of serum amylase and alkaline phosphatase estimation.	111	77	J05
20. Diagnostic significance of serum alkaline phosphatase.	111	74	D15
21. Write the diagnostic significance of each of the following enzymes: a. Lipase b. Alanine amino transferase c. Creatine kinase	111	77, 262	J21(RS4)
22. Define isoenzymes. Give one example.	112	75	D05, J06, J08
23. Name the isoenzymes of LDH. Mention their significance.	112	75	D03
24. CPK isoenzymes and its clinical significance.	114	262	J99, J07, J15

Contd...

Contd...

	STNRN	VSDN	
25. Explain troponin as a marker for myocardial infarction.	115	262	D05(RS2)
26. Explain enzyme profile in myocardial infarction.	115	262	J07(RS2)
27. Write the type of inhibitions seen in the following:			F21(RS4)
a. Inhibition of vitamin K by dicoumarol—an anticoagulant	a. 95	a. 69	
b. Inhibition of cyclo-oxygenase by aspirin	b. 97	b. 71	
c. Inhibition of placental alkaline phosphatase by phenylalanine	c.—	c. —	
Multiple Choice Questions			
1. 5'-Nucleotidase is more specific for: a. Myocardial infarction b. Prostate cancer c. **Obstructive liver disease** d. Wilson's disease	110	77	J21(RS4)
2. Serum acid phosphatase enzyme is increased in: a. Hepatic disease b. Myocardial infarction c. Muscle disease d. **Prostate cancer**	111	78	J21(RS4)
CHAPTER 7: VITAMINS			
Long Essays			
1. Give an account on chemistry, sources, absorption, daily requirement, biochemical functions, manifestations of deficiency and toxic effects of vitamin A.	122	513	D09(RS2), D98, D03, J06
2. Answer the following: a. Which vitamin is called sunshine vitamin? b. What is its active form? c. How it is formed? d. Write the biochemical functions and deficiency manifestations of this vitamin.	127	519	J21(RS4)
3. How provitamin D is converted to its active form? Give an account of chemistry, sources, daily requirement, biochemical functions and deficiency manifestations of vitamin D.	127	519	J03

Contd...

Contd...

	STNRN	VSDN	
4. Discuss the chemistry, source, requirement, metabolic functions and deficiency manifestations of vitamin C (ascorbic acid) in the human body.	135	548	D05(RS2), D99
5. What are the sources, functions, deficiency manifestations and daily recommended allowance of thiamine?	138	531	D17(RS3), D09
6. Name the coenzyme forms of vitamin involved in amino acid metabolism. Discuss the biochemical functions and deficiency manifestations of this vitamin.	146	536	J06(RS2)
7. Discuss RDA, Functions and deficiency manifestations of folic acid. How is it interlinked to vitamin B_{12}?	154, 160	540	D16(RS3)
Short Essays			
1. Name a provitamin form of vitamin A. Add a note on sources, biochemical functions, daily requirement, causes and features of deficiency of vitamin A.	122	513	J09(RS2), J10(RS2), D11(RS3), J12(RS3), J18(RS3), N20(RS3), D02, J05, J09
2. A 10-year-old boy had difficulty in vision at night. However, his vision was quite normal during daytime except when he entered a dimly lit room. On investigation, his plasma retinol levels were found to be low: a. Suggest the probable diagnosis. Which nutrient deficiency causes this disease? b. Enumerate any four functions of the nutrient. c. Explain Wald's visual cycle.	126	514	F21(RS4)
3. Wald's visual cycle.	124	514	J08
4. Active form of vitamin D and its biochemical role.	127	519	D08
5. Vitamin D metabolism. Add a brief note hepatic osteodystrophy.	127	519	D05
6. Synthesis of calcitriol in the body and its uses.	127	519	J00
7. Biochemical functions and causes and features of deficiency of vitamin D.	128	514	J07(RS2), J11(RS2), J04

Contd...

Contd...

	STNRN	VSDN	
8. Vitamin E.	131	523	J99, D04
9. Sources, daily requirements, functions and deficiency manifestation of vitamin C.	135	548	D07(RS2), J08(RS2), D18(RS3), D07, D11
10. Explain the following aspects of thiamine: (a) Coenzyme form, (b) Biochemical function and (c) Deficiency.	138	531	J05(RS2), D01, D14
11. Mention the functions of thiamine pyrophosphate (TTP) citing the reactions in which it is involved.	138	531	J14
12. Explain the following aspects of riboflavin: (a) Coenzyme forms, (b) Biochemical functions.	140	532	D02
13. Give the biochemical functions of niacin with examples and manifestation of its deficiency.	143	534	J13(RS3)
14. Name the coenzyme form of vitamin B_6 (pyridoxine). Describe the biochemical reactions involving it/biochemical functions of pyridoxine (pyridoxal phosphate co-decarboxylase).	146	536	D10(RS2), D98, J02, D14
15. Give the coenzyme role of pantothenic acid and its importance.	152	538	J15(RS3)
16. Chemistry, sources, daily requirement, coenzyme forms and functions of folic acid.	153	540	D06(RS2), J04
17. Hyperhomocysteinemia.	156	542	J07
18. Coenzymes of cobalamin and its functions.	156	543	J19(RS3)
19. Coenzyme form of vitamin B_{12} and its biochemical functions.	157	543	D15(RS3)
Short Answers			
1. Hypervitaminosis.	—	519, 525, 524	J09
2. FIGLU excretion test.	—	542	J13(RS3), D15
3. Provitamins.	—	519	J17(RS3), D00
4. Vitamin A—functions (antioxidant role), RDA, deficiency manifestations.	124	514	D08(RS2), J01, D04, D10, J11, D16
5. Visual cycle.	124	515	J00
6. Mention causes and clinical features of hypervitaminosis A.	126	519	J14

Contd...

Contd...

	STNRN	VSDN	
7. Vitamin D—biochemical functions, deficiency symptoms.	128	519	D00
8. Vitamin E—functions/antioxidant role.	131	523	J06(RS2), J15, D15
9. Vitamin K—biochemical role and requirement.	133	524	J12(RS3), D15(RS3), J02, J05, J10, J14
10. Vitamin C—functions (role in iron absorption), deficiency manifestations (scurvy).	136	548	D10(RS2), J19(RS3), J09, J12
11. Thiamine—sources, daily requirements, role, deficiency manifestations.	138	531	D99, D05, J06, D10, J11
12. TPP as a coenzyme in two metabolic reaction of the body.	138	531	J00
13. Types and causes of beri-beri.	139	531	J12(RS3), J11(RS2), D11
14. What is the coenzymic form of niacin and give one reaction where it is utilized?	143	534	D06
15. Niacin—coenzymic forms and deficiency manifestations (pellagra).	143	534	J17(RS3), J00, D14, D15
16. Pellagra.	144	535	N20(RS3)
17. What is the coenzyme form of pyridoxine? Write two pyridoxine dependent reactions.	146	534	F21(RS4)
18. Functions of pyridoxal phosphate.	146	536	J07(RS2)
19. Which vitamin deficiency is likely to develop in patients on isoniazid, an antitubercular drug? What is the co-enzyme form of this vitamin? Write one biochemical reaction dependent on this nutrient.	149	536	J21(RS4)
20. How is histamine formed? What is the role of histamine?	147	343	J10
21. Biotin.	150	539	D00
22. Name the anti-egg white injury factor, its source and coenzyme function	150	539	J01, D04
23. Describe two carboxylation reactions.	150	539	J05, J08
24. Functions of folic acid.	154	540	J00
25. Explain the role of folic acid in DNA synthesis.	154	542	D16

Contd...

Contd...

	STNRN	VSDN	
26. FIGLU.	155	542	J14(RS3), D98, D00
27. Name two folate antagonists and their therapeutic use.	156	543	D02
28. What are the coenzymic forms of cobalamin?	156	543	D05
29. Name the biochemical functions of vitamin B_{12}.	157	544	D01
30. Vitamin B_{12} deficiency—causes and biochemical explanations	159	544	D19(RS3)
31. What are antivitamins? Give two examples (vitamin antagonists).	162	540, 542	J03, D08
32. Mention the functions of vitamin E and vitamin K.	132, 134	523, 524	J04
33. Cause of scurvy and beri-beri.	137, 139	531, 548	J13(RS3)
34. Write coenzyme forms of niacin and riboflavin.	143, 140	533, 534	D00
35. Coenzyme form of niacin and folic acid.	143, 154	534, 540	D08
36. Coenzymic form of vitamin B_{12} and folic acid.	156, 154	540, 543	D11
37. What is the daily requirement of thiamine, niacin and pyridoxine?	138, 144, 149	531, 534	J09(RS2)

SECTION 2: PHYSIOLOGICAL BIOCHEMISTRY

CHAPTER 8: DIGESTION AND ABSORPTION

Long Essay

1. Write in detail about the digestion and absorption of lipids? Write about causes of fatty stools.	174	220	J98

Short Essays

1. Give an account of digestion of carbohydrates from GIT.	168	146	D13
2. Explain the mechanism involved in the absorption of glucose. Describe the causes and features of lactose intolerance.	170	146	J99, J02, D04
3. Lactose intolerance.	171	147	D05

Contd...

BIOCHEMISTRY

Contd...

	STNRN	VSDN	
4. Write in brief about the digestion and absorption of proteins.	171	289	D14(RS3), J06, J13
5. Digestion and absorption of lipids.	174	220	D15(RS3), D19(RS3), J12
6. Enzymes involved in the digestion of lipids (lipases).	174	220	D05
7. Name the different types of lipases involved in lipid metabolism. Mention their sites of action, function and activation.	174	221	J03
Short Answers			
1. Name the enzymes involved in carbohydrate digestion.	168	146	D09
2. Digestion and absorption of disaccharides.	168	146	D12(RS3)
3. Describe the absorption of glucose.	169	146	J04
4. Lactose intolerance—causes and features.	171	147	D98, D99, J04, D08, J12
5. Give an example of proteolytic enzyme and its specificity.	171	289	D06, D14
6. Name the two endopeptidases with their specifications.	171	289	J09(RS2)
7. Role of hydrochloric acid in protein digestion.	172	289	J01, D04
8. How is pepsinogen activated? What is the function of pepsin?	172	289	J10
9. Pepsinogen activation and action of trypsin.	172	289	D11
10. Describe the role of bile salts in lipid metabolism.	174	220	J13
11. What is steatorrhea? Mention the causes.	177	223	J12(RS3), J02, J03, D16
CHAPTER 9: PLASMA PROTEINS			
Long Essay			
1. What are plasma proteins? Write a note on their separation and functions.	182	444	D08
Short Essays			
1. How plasma proteins are separated? Explain the significance of M band. What is A/G ratio? What is its clinical significance?	182	444	J04
2. What is electrophoresis? Name five plasma proteins and their functions.	182	444	D11

Contd...

Contd...

	STNRN	VSDN	
3. Name and explain the functions of plasma proteins with clinical significance.	183	445	D14(RS3)
4. What is normal serum protein level? Mention three important functions of albumin.	183	445	D12(RS3)
5. Enumerate the functions of albumin. Mention the causes of hypoalbuminemia and consequences of hypoalbuminemia.	183	446	J11(RS2), J03
6. List conditions when albumin/globulin (A/G) ratio is altered.	183	447	D12(RS3)
7. Transport proteins of blood.	184	448	J09(RS2)
8. A 40-year-old male came with the complaints of difficulty in breathing, shortness of breath and tightness of chest. History revealed that he is chronic smoker for the past 15 years. Chest X-ray and CT scan showed changes suggestive of emphysema. a. Deficiency of which plasma protein causes this condition. b. Explain the biochemical basis of emphysema in smokers. c. Name any two serine proteases.	185	450	J21(RS4)
9. Acute phase proteins.	186	449	J10(RS2)
10. Immunoglobulins—enumerate, structure and functions.	187	744	N20(RS3), J03, D12, D16
Short Answers			
1. What is the normal level of plasma proteins? Name a disease which features hypoalbuminemia.	—	445, 447	D05
2. Negative acute phase reactants.	—	450	D15
3. Describe how plasma protein are separated in the clinical laboratory.	182	444	D17(RS3)
4. What is electrophoresis? Enumerate major classes of proteins separated on electrophoresis.	182	444	J01, D04
5. Mention the normal albumin/globulin (A/G) ratio. Give two disorders associated with altered A/G ratio.	183	447	F21(RS4)
6. Serum albumin—functions.	183	447	D06(RS2), J10
7. Normal values of serum proteins and its fractions.	184	446	J99

Contd...

BIOCHEMISTRY

Contd...

	STNRN	VSDN	
8. Plasma proteins—enumerate and functions of plasma proteins.	184	446	J16(RS3), J06, D10, D12
9. Hypoalbuminemia.	185	447	D17(RS3)
10. Ceruloplasmin.	186	449	J99, D00, J09, J15
11. Acute phase proteins.	186	449	D18(RS3)
12. Immunoglobulins—enumerate, structure and functions. Outline the structure of immunoglobulins.	187	744	D10(RS2), D12(RS3), J18(RS3), D07, J08, D10
13. Immunoglobin G (IgG).	188	745	J98
14. Immunoglobulin A (IgA) and immunoglobulin M (IgM).	188	746	J11(RS2)
15. Structure of immunoglobulin M.	189	746	J14
16. Bence-Jones proteins—significance and detection.	190	747	D05(RS2), J06(RS2), D11(RS3), D01, D08
17. Anticoagulants.	192	454	J08(RS2)

CHAPTER 10: HEMOGLOBIN AND PORPHYRIA

Long Essays

1. Explain in detail the reactions of heme synthesis? Name the regulatory enzyme of this pathway. How is it regulated?	208	377	J21(RS4)
2. Outline heme synthesis. Write a note on its function and abnormal hemoglobin.	208	377, 396	J09
3. Describe the synthesis and breakdown of hemoglobin. Write a note on hemoglobinopathies.	208, 201, 213	377, 396	D13(RS3)

Short Essays

1. Name five heme proteins and their functions.	—	376	D08(RS2)
2. What is methemoglobin? How it is formed? Mention the causes for methemoglobinemia. How it is detected?	201	394	J16(RS3), D99
3. Name the different types of hemoglobin variants indicating their defects/ hemoglobinopathies (abnormal hemoglobins).	201	396	D19(RS3), D05(RS2)
4. Sickle cell hemoglobin.	201	396	J98

Contd...

Contd...

	STNRN	VSDN	
5. Discuss the manifestations, molecular basis and laboratory diagnosis of sickle cell disease. What is the biological advantage of sickle cell trait?	202	396	J01
6. A 8-year-old girl from endemic malaria area who had splenomegaly was investigated for routine hematology, which revealed low hemoglobin of 7 g%. Peripheral smear revealed crescent shaped RBCs. She had no history of malaria attack. a. What could be the molecular defect of hemoglobin in the above case. b. Name the biochemical investigations which can be done to confirm the diagnosis. c. Reason out why these patients show resistance to malaria.	204	397	F21(RS4)
7. Heme synthesis (regulation).	208	377	J17(RS3), J18(RS3), N20(RS3), D00, D11
8. Porphyrias—causes and general features.	210	379	J17(RS3), J18(RS3), N20(RS3), D00, D11
9. What are porphyrias? How are they classified? Name the enzymatic defect and biochemical findings in any one/four of the porphyrias.	210	379	J15(RS3), J00, J03
10. What is porphyria? Mention the defect, signs and symptoms of acute intermittent porphyria.	210	379	D09(RS2), D11(RS3)
11. Congenital erythropoietic porphyria.	212	381	J99, D04
12. Catabolism (degradation) of heme (hemoglobin) in the body adding a note on clinical significance.	213	383	F21(RS4), D07(RS2), D14(RS3), D98, J00, D01, D08
13. Bile pigments (bilirubin)—describe the metabolism (formation, transport and detoxification). Write the normal values of serum bilirubin. Name the abnormalities associated with bilirubin metabolism.	213	383	J07(RS2), J09(RS2), J14(RS3), J16(RS3), J99, D04, J14, D14

Contd...

Contd...

	STNRN	VSDN	
14. Jaundice.	215	386	D12
15. Hemolytic jaundice.	215	386	D99
16. Unconjugated hyperbilirubinemia.	215	386	D08(RS2)
17. Hepatocellular jaundice.	215	387	D09
18. Interpret the following Liver function tests report: (a) Total bilirubin: 7.7 mg/dL; (b) Direct bilirubin: 3.6 mg/dL; (c) Alkaline phosphatase: 265 IU/L; (d) Ehrlich's test: Negative; (e) Stool sample: Clay color. a. What is the probable diagnosis? b. Mention the possible causes for the above condition. c. Substantiate with reasons for increase in conjugated fraction of bilirubin.	215	387	F21(RS4)
Short Answers			
1. What is Dubin-Johnson disease?	—	386	J01, D04
2. What is the effect of pH and pCO_2 on the oxygen dissociation curve?	198	389	D09
3. Hemoglobin as buffering agent.	198	389	D15(RS3)
4. 2,3-bisphosphoglycerate.	199	392	J06(RS2)
5. Carboxy hemoglobin.	201	394	J08(RS2), J99
6. Methemoglobin.	201	394	J10(RS2)
7. Name the hemoglobinopathies (abnormal hemoglobins).	201	396	D07, D09
8. Sickle cell hemoglobin—biochemical defects, alteration in function.	201	397	J06, J07, D13
9. Sickle cell anemia—causes, molecular defect and consequences.	202	397	D07(RS2), J11(RS2), D08, D12
10. Biochemical defect in thalassemia.	205	399	J13(RS3)
11. Name the levels at which heme synthesis is regulated.	210	377	D02, D07
12. What porphyrias? Name one disorder indicating the underlying cause.	210	379	J04
13. Explain any two types of porphyrias.	210	379	D10
14. Acute intermittent porphyria.	210	379	J14(RS3), J18(RS3), D99, D13

Contd...

BIOCHEMISTRY

Contd...

	STNRN	VSDN	
15. Name two porphyrias and the enzyme defect in them.	211	379	J08
16. Degradation of heme.	213	383	J05(RS2), D06(RS2), J04
17. How is bilirubin conjugated (made water soluble).	214	384	J06(RS2)
18. Fate of bilirubin.	215	384	D15
19. Name two causes of unconjugated hyperbilirubinemia.	215	386	J07
20. Normal level of total bilirubin in serum. What is conjugated bilirubin?	215	385	D99, D06
21. Define jaundice. Mention one cause for different types of jaundice.	215	386	D03
22. Obstructive jaundice and its diagnosis (biochemical findings—serum and urine)..	215	387	J21(RS4), D13(RS3), J02, D08
23. Physiological jaundice.	216	386	J11
24. Name two congenital hyperbilirubinemias and defect in each of them.	216	386	D01
25. What is Crigler-Najjar syndrome? Name the enzymatic defect.	216	386	D02, D05
26. Give enzyme defect in the following conditions.			
a. Drug-induced hemolytic anemia.	a. —	a. —	J09(RS2)
b. Criggler-Najjar syndrome.	b. 216	b. 386	J14(RS3)
27. Gilberts syndrome.	216	386	J14(RS3)
Multiple Choice Questions			
1. The enzyme defect in acute intermittent porphyria: a. **PBG-deaminase** b. UPG-cosynthase c. Ferrochelatase d. UPG-decarboxylase	210	379	J21(RS4)

CHAPTER 11: BIOLOGICAL OXIDATION

Long Essays

1. Describe the components of electron transport chain. Write a note on uncouplers and inhibitors.	223, 230	131, 138	D08
2. Discuss in detail oxidative phosphorylation and enumerate its inhibitors.	226	128, 138	J10(RS2)

Contd...

BIOCHEMISTRY

Contd...

	STNRN	VSDN	
Short Essays			
1. Write the different components of electron transport chain. Draw a neatly labeled diagram of the complexes of the electron transport chain. Mention four inhibitors of ETC/ Name any two site-specific inhibitors of each complex.	224	131	J21(RS4), J14(RS3), D16
2. Describe the single electron carrier components of respiratory chain. Indicate the sites of ATP formation during electron transport. Name two inhibitors of electron transport.	224	131	J07(RS2), D07(RS2), D02, J03, D03, J08, J10, J13
3. What are cytochromes? Indicate their location and functions.	226	129	D99
4. What is oxidative phosphorylation? Explain its mechanism (chemiosmotic theory). Mention inhibitors and uncouplers of oxidative phosphorylation.	226	128	F21(RS4), J05(RS2), J06(RS2), D19(RS3), D98, J01, J04, J06, D06, J14, D14, D15
5. What is P:O ratio? Which are inhibitors of electron transport chain?	227	128	D05(RS2)
6. What are uncouplers? Mention the uncouplers of oxidative phosphorylation.	231	128	J16(RS3), J15
7. Shuttle systems to transport extra-mitochondrial reducing equivalents.	232	132	D05
8. Classify the enzymes of biological oxidation. Give one example for each.	234	128	D01
Short Answers			
1. Differentiate between uncoupler and inhibitors.	—	—	D16
2. Expand ATP. What is its free energy of hydrolysis?	219	130	D11
3. High energy (phosphate) compounds.	220	130	J13(RS3), J02, D16
4. Components of electron transport chain.	224	131	J17(RS3), D11

Contd...

BIOCHEMISTRY

Contd...

	STNRN	VSDN	
5. Diagrammatic representation of mitochondrial electron transport chain and location of ATP formation sites.	225	132	D09(RS2)
6. Cytochromes.	226	129	D11(RS3)
7. Oxidative phosphorylation—mechanism (chemiosmotic theory), inhibitors, uncouplers (with two examples).	226	138	D06(RS2), J08(RS2), J11(RS2), J15(RS3), D17(RS3), D18(RS3), J98, J03, J05, D12, D13, D16
8. P:O ratio.	227	134	J09, D09, J11
9. Name the inhibitors of cytochrome oxidase.	230	134	D06
10. Site specific inhibitors of electron transport chain with one example for each site.	230	134	D16(RS3), J19(RS3)
11. Ionophores.	231	22	D12(RS3)
12. Mitochondrial shuttle systems.	232	132	J13(RS3)
13. Describe malate—aspartate shuttle. What is its significance?	233	132	J01, D04

Multiple Choice Questions

1. _____ is known to act as a physiological uncoupler. a. Valinomysin b. **Thyroxine** c. Carboxine d. Oligomycin	231	134	J21(RS4)

SECTION 3: METABOLISM

CHAPTER 12: INTRODUCTION TO METABOLISM

None

CHAPTER 13: METABOLISM OF CARBOHYDRATES

Long Essays

1. Describe the reactions of glycolysis indicating the enzymes. Add a note on net yield of ATP under aerobic and anaerobic conditions.	244	149	D17(RS3)

Contd...

Contd...

	STNRN	VSDN	
2. Give a detailed account on glycolysis. Explain the energetics and regulation of this pathway. What is the significance of Rapaport-Leubering cycle?	244, 251	149, 156	J98, J08, D12
3. Describe the process of aerobic glycolysis. What is substrate level phosphorylation? What is the effect of insulin and cortisol on blood glucose level?	244, 648	127, 149, 189	D11
4. Why TCA cycle is called as common metabolic pathway? Describe in detail the tricarboxylic acid cycle (Kreb's citric acid cycle), energy production and its significance. How is it regulated? What is its amphibolic role? Explain how carbohydrates, lipids and amino acids enter this cycle.	253	120	J08(RS2), D13(RS2), J04, J10, D14
5. Describe in detail the major catabolic pathway for acetyl CoA in aerobic organisms. How does it play a pivotal role in metabolism?	253	120	D05
6. What is gluconeogenesis? Write in detail about gluconeogenesis in humans from its predominant precursor (conversion of lactate to glucose) and mention its significance. Write about glucose alanine cycle.	258	158, 160	D11(RS3), D98, D00, J03
7. Discuss the formation of glucose from noncarbohydrate substances.	258	158	J15
8. What is gluconeogenesis? Trace the pathway of gluconeogenesis starting from alanine. Mention the key enzymes and how they are regulated.	258, 261	158	J09(RS2), D19(RS3)
9. Discuss about the metabolism of glycogen.	263	162	J99
10. What is the biomedical importance of muscle and liver glycogen? Describe the process of glycogen synthesis with its regulation. Name two glycogen storage diseases.	263	162, 166	D06, J11
11. Define glycogenesis and glycogenolysis. Write the reactions of glycogenesis and glycogenolysis in liver. How are these two pathways reciprocally regulated?	263	162, 166	J07(RS2)

Contd...

Contd...

	STNRN	VSDN	
12. Describe the reactions of pentose phosphate pathway (hexose monophosphate shunt). Why is it called multifunctional? Mention the significance of this pathway.	269	166	J02, J09, D10, D15
Short Essays			
1. What is the difference between oxidative and substrate level phosphorylation? Give two examples of substrate level phosphorylation with complete reaction.	—	127	D10(RS2), J13(RS3), D14(RS3), J99, D04
2. How is glycogen digested and absorbed? Describe glycogenolysis in the liver.	168, 265	146, 162	J15(RS3)
3. Glucose transporters.	243	147	D06
4. Regulation of glycolysis.	249	153	J07
5. Discuss the Embden-Meyerhof pathway that occurs in RBC. Add a note on its energetics.	251	156	J14(RS3)
6. 2,3-biphosphoglycerate pathway in erythrocytes (Rapaport-Leubering cycle).	251	156	J10(RS2), D10(RS2), D06
7. Fate of pyruvate.	251	156	D06
8. Pyruvate oxidation.	251	156	J99, D04
9. Pyruvate dehydrogenase complex—enzymes and co-enzymes components, mechanism of action and biomedical importance.	252	156	D07(RS2), J12
10. Citric acid (TCA) cycle—reactions, energy releasing steps, energetic, amphibolic role.	253	120	J09(RS2), D11(RS3), J12(RS3), J18(RS3), N20(RS3), J06, J13
11. Define anaplerosis. Describe any four anaplerotic reactions of citric acid cycle intermediates.	257	125	J21(RS4)
12. Gluconeogenesis—(key) reactions (from lactate/alanine), key enzymes, significance.	258	158	D05(RS2), J06(RS2), J13(RS3), D16(RS3), D02, D05, D08, D09, D16
13. What is fate of lactate produced in the muscle? Explain the reactions.	261	161	J01

Contd...

Contd...

	STNRN	VSDN	
14. Cori's cycle.	261	155	J12(RS3), J14
15. Glucose alanine cycle.	261	160	J08
16. Synthesis of glycogen (glycogenesis)—reactions and its significance.	263	163	J08(RS2), D07, J12, D13
17. Glycogenolysis—reactions, regulation.	265	162	J10(RS2), J11(RS2), J16(RS3), D18(RS3), J02, D02, J05
18. Glycogen storage disease.	269	166	D06(RS2), J17(RS3), J00, J03, J06, J14
19. A 5-year-old girl was brought to the hospital with enlarged abdomen. History revealed that her childhood development was comparatively slow, frequently hungry, lethargic and irritable. Clinical examination showed enlarged liver. Biochemical investigations of blood sample revealed reduced fasting blood glucose levels and elevated levels of serum lactate, triglyceride and uric acid. a. Suggest the probable diagnosis. b. Name the enzyme defect. c. What is the biochemical basis for fasting hypoglycemia, lactic acidosis and hyperuricemia in this condition.	269	166	F21(RS4)
20. Hexose monophosphate shunt—reactions (oxidative phase), significance.	269	166	D13(RS3), J17(RS3), D18(RS3), D06
21. Uronic acid pathway.	275	171	J13
22. How is galactose metabolized? Add a note on galactosemia.	277	209	N20(RS3), D00, D07
23. Metabolism of fructose.	278	207	J00
24. Fructose intolerance.	280	208	D98
Short Answers			
1. Explain substrate level phosphorylation with two examples.	—	127	D01, D02, D07, J11, J12
2. Give the significance of uronic acid pathway.	—	171	J09(RS2)
3. Aldolase B.	—	208	D00

Contd...

Contd...

	STNRN	VSDN	
4. What are the major differences between hexokinase and glucokinase?	245	153	J05
5. Glucokinase.	245	153	D99
6. Energetics in aerobic and anaerobic pathway of EM pathway (glucose oxidation).	248	149	D99, J09
7. Regulation of glycolysis at the phosphofructokinase step.	249	153	J18(RS3)
8. What is the end product of aerobic glycolysis? Illustrate the fate of this compound.	251	156	J21(RS4)
9. Write short note on Rapaport-Leubering cycle.	251	156	J16(RS3), D17(RS3), D12
10. Conversion of pyruvate to acetyl CoA.	251	156	J06
11. Pyruvate dehydrogenase complex.	252	156	J14(RS3), D18(RS3)
12. Amphibolic role of citric acid cycle.	257	125	D10
13. Anapleurotic reactions of citric acid cycle for three intermediates.	257	125	J19(RS3), J00, D00, J03
14. Any three enzymes unique (key) to gluconeogenesis.	259	158	J11(RS2), J13
15. Cori's cycle.	261	155	J11
16. Describe glucose alanine cycle. Mention its significance.	261	160	J01, D01, D04
17. Glycogen storage disorders.	269	166	J13(RS3)
18. Von Gierke's disease.	269	166	D17(RS3), D99
19. Muscle phosphorylase deficiency.	271	167	D98
20. Mention significance of HMP shunt pathway.	272	167	D05(RS2), J08(RS2), J08, J12
21. Glucose-6-phosphate dehydrogenase deficiency.	275	166	D07(RS2)
22. Uridine diphosphate glucose—glucuronic acid.	276	171	J15(RS3)
23. Galactosemia—enzyme defect, clinical features and biochemical findings.	278	209	D16(RS3), J18(RS3), D99, D02, J05, D12, D16

Contd...

Contd...

	STNRN	VSDN	
24. What is the sorbitol pathway? Write the significance of sorbitol pathway.	279	171	J21(RS4)
25. Aldolase B deficiency.	280	208	J98
26. Name the enzyme defective in galactosemia and hereditary fructose intolerance.	278, 280	208, 209	J02, D06
Multiple Choice Questions			
1. Glucose transporter 4 is the major glucose transporter in: a. RBC b. Neurons c. **Adipose tissue** d. Intestine	244	147	J21(RS4)
CHAPTER 14: METABOLISM OF LIPIDS			
Long Essays			
1. What is carnitine and its role in oxidation of fatty acids? Enumerate the steps of beta oxidation of saturated fatty acids (palmitic acid). Write a note on energetic of palmitic acid. Explain the regulation of acetyl CoA in our body.	288	224	D08(RS2), J15(RS3), J01, D02, D04, J05, J06, D07, D10, D13, J15
2. A 25-years-old patient known cases of type 1 diabetes, was brought to casualty in comatose state. History revealed that he was not taking insulin regularly. Biochemical analysis of blood and urine showed the following findings: (a) Blood sugar—510 mg/dL; (b) Urine for Rothera's test and Benedict's test—positive; (c) Blood gas analysis report showed pH—7.2; (d) Bicarbonate—12 mEq/L. a. Suggest your probable diagnosis. b. Name the compounds which give Rothera's test positive. c. Explain the principle of Rothera's test. d. Explain the steps of synthesis, utilization of these compounds.	295	237	J21(RS4)
3. Describe the formation (ketogenesis), utilization (ketolysis) and clinical significance of ketone bodies (ketosis).	295	236	J11(RS2), J18(RS3), J11

Contd...

Contd...

	STNRN	VSDN	
4. What is ketosis? What are the causes? What are ketone bodies? Enumerate the steps of formation and utilization of ketone bodies?	295	236	J00
5. Name the ketone bodies. Give two conditions characterized by excessive production of ketone bodies. Explain the metabolic derangements and consequences of ketosis.	295	236	J05(RS2)
6. Describe in detail the de novo synthesis of fatty acids. Add a note on short- and long-term mechanisms that regulate lipogenesis.	298	228	J07
7. Give an account of cholesterol biosynthesis with its regulation. Add a note on atherosclerosis.	311	233, 244	J16(RS3)
8. What are lipoproteins? How are they classified? How are chylomicrons metabolized?	319	251	D09
9. Classify plasma lipoproteins, explain their composition, transport and functions.	319	251	J13(RS3)
10. Define lipoproteins. Mention the different lipoproteins involved in transport of lipids. Explain metabolism of dietary lipids under the following headings: (a) Assembly of dietary lipids; (b) Transport; (c) Utilization in peripheral tissues; (d) Metabolic rate.	319	251	F21(RS4)
Short Essays			
1. List various types of fatty acid oxidation. Write about activation of fatty acids for oxidation.	288	223	D07(RS2), J07
2. Describe the beta oxidation of fatty acids. Add a note on energetics of palmitic acid oxidation.	288	223	D05(RS2), D14(RS3), D16(RS3), D19(RS3) D05, J09
3. Explain how odd chain fatty acids are oxidized.	293	225	J14
4. Metabolic activity and abnormality in peroxisomes.	293	—	D05

Contd...

BIOCHEMISTRY

Contd...

	STNRN	VSDN	
5. Ketone bodies—enumerate, formation (ketogenesis), utilization (ketolysis), clinical significance (ketosis).	295	236	J06(RS2), D09(RS2), N20(RS3), D00, D06, J09, D12, D14
6. Ketosis.	296	236	J08
7. Outline the de novo synthesis of fatty acid. What are the advantages of having a multifunctional enzyme complex?	298	228	D13(RS3)
8. Fatty acid synthase complex.	299	228	J11(RS2), D06, J09
9. Mention the defect and clinical features of four lipid storage disorder.	310	284	D16
10. Name the ring structure present in cholesterol. Write the key regulatory step in the synthesis of cholesterol. Name four compounds derived from cholesterol.	39, 313, 315	244	D17(RS3)
11. Outline the steps for synthesis of cholesterol. Discuss the rate limiting step and regulation of synthesis of cholesterol.	311	244	D11(RS3), J18 (RS3)
12. How is HMG CoA formed? What is its importance?	311	245	D13
13. Catabolic products of cholesterol. Describe the biomedical importance of three derivatives of cholesterol.	315	247	J09(RS2), D10(RS2), J98, J03
14. How are bile acid synthesized? Mention two functions of bile acids.	315	255	J15(RS3), D10
15. Lipoproteins—enumerate, composition and functions.	319	251	J05(RS2), J14(RS3), J02, D02, D03, J06, J10
16. Chylomicrons (metabolism).	319	250	J10(RS2)
17. Give an account of metabolism of LDL.	321	251	D13
18. Metabolism of high-density lipoprotein and its significance.	322	252	N20(RS3)
19. Fatty liver (causes) and lipotrophic factors.	324	234	D06(RS2), J07(RS2), D08(RS2), D14(RS3), J19(RS3), D07, D08, J13, D15
Short Answers			
1. Enumerate the consequences of obesity.	—	592	J11

Contd...

Contd...

	STNRN	VSDN	
2. What is the significance of brown adipose tissue?	—	234	J04
3. What is carnitine? Mention its biochemical role of carnitine in β-oxidation (carnitine cycle).	289	224	J06(RS2), J02, J12, J13, D13, D14
4. Explain how long chain fatty acid are transported into the mitochondria.	289	224	J21(RS4)
5. Energetics in the oxidation of one molecule of palmitic acid to carbon dioxide and water.	291	226	J18(RS3)
6. Methyl malonyl aciduria.	293	227	D98
7. Give enzyme defect in the methyl malonyl aciduria and homocystinuria.	293, 364	227, 346	D16
8. Mention how propionyl CoA is formed during fatty acid oxidation.	293	227	J00
9. Refsum's disease.	294	228	J08(RS2)
10. Ketone bodies.	295	236	D08
11. Name the ketone bodies. Mention two causes of ketosis.	295	236	D02, J03, J04
12. Ketosis.	296	236	J17(RS3)
13. Niemann-Pick disease.	309	283	J10(RS2)
14. Name two lipid storage disorders and indicate the corresponding enzyme defect.	310	283	D07
15. Name four substances synthesized from cholesterol.	315	247	D06
16. Name bile acids. How are they formed?	315	255	J10
17. Bile salts—enumerate, functions (role in digestion).	315	255	J99, J05, D08, D09, D11, J12
18. Reverse cholesterol transport.	316	254	J15(RS3), D05
19. What is normal serum level of cholesterol? Name its four biological functions.	316	244	J07(RS2)
20. What is the normal level of serum cholesterol? Name one bile acid formed from cholesterol.	316	244	J07
21. Plasma lipoproteins—enumerate, functions.	319	251	J17(RS3), D98, J08, D12
22. HDL cholesterol.	319	248	D99, J12
23. What are functions of apolipoproteins?	319	249	J09(RS2)

Contd...

Contd...

	STNRN	VSDN	
24. Name the cholesterol rich lipoproteins.	320	252	D06
25. Justify the role of HDL as scavenger of cholesterol.	322	254	D00
26. Fatty liver—causes.	324	234	J00, D03, J06, J12, J14
27. Lipotropic factors.	326	235	J98, J13, D14
28. Mention two inborn errors of lipid metabolism and indicate the enzyme defect.	306, 309	283	D03
29. Name the biochemical defect in: a. Niemann-Pick disease. b. Gauchers's disease.	306, 309	283	J03
Multiple Choice Questions			
1. The site of action of hormone sensitive lipase is in: a. Small intestine b. Capillary walls c. Mouth d. **Adipocytes**	286	232	J21(RS4)
2. Which one of the lipoprotein fraction is elevated in hyperlipoproteinemia type IIA? a. VLDL b. **LDL** c. HDL d. Chylomicrons	323	251	J21(RS4)
CHAPTER 15: METABOLISM OF AMINO ACIDS			
Long Essays			
1. Describe how ammonia is formed (sources of ammonia) in the body? Add a note on its transportation. Describe how ammonia is detoxified in the body and name two inborn errors associated with this process.	336	294	D18(RS3), D01, J05, D06, J12, D16
2. Describe in detail the steps of urea cycle. How is it linked to TCA cycle? What is the reference range for serum urea? Write the causes of uremia.	338	297, 301	D11(RS3)
3. Describe the urea cycle. What is the normal blood urea level? Name two conditions in which blood urea level increases.	338	297, 301	D02

Contd...

BIOCHEMISTRY

Contd...

	STNRN	VSDN	
4. Describe the metabolism, metabolic defects and special products formed from glycine giving their biomedical importance. Why is glycine nutritionally nonessential?	343	307	D05(RS2), J02, J04, D07
5. How is creatinine synthesized? Discuss about creatinine clearance and its clinical significance.	345	309	J99
6. Name the aromatic amino acids. What are biologically important compounds derived from tyrosine? Describe the metabolism of phenylalanine and tyrosine. Outline the synthesis of different products obtained from phenylalanine. Discuss the inborn errors associated with metabolism (tyrosinemia/alkaptonuria).	347	332	D10(RS2), J12(RS3), J17(RS3), N20(RS3), D99, J01, D04, J07, J08, J10
7. A 5-year-old boy was brought to a pediatrician with history of mousy odor of urine and delay in achieving cognitive functions. On examination, the boy's skin and hair was fair in color with hypopigmentation. a. What is the probable diagnosis? b. Name the enzyme defect in the above disorder. c. Write the pathway for catabolism of the above amino acid. d. Mention the reason for the cause of mousy odor in urine. e. What biochemical tests are done to confirm the diagnosis?	352	336	F21(RS4)
8. A 6-year-old child was brought to the OPD with complaints of mental retardation, delayed development milestones, hyperactive and seizures. The child had light colored hair, skin and unpleasant mousy body odor. Serum phenylalanine was 35 mg/dL (normal 1–2 mg/dL). Ferric chloride test showed transient blue-green color in urine. a. Suggest the probable diagnosis. b. Mention the enzyme defect and write the reaction catalyzed by their enzyme.	352	336	J21(RS4)

Contd...

Contd...

	STNRN	VSDN	
c. Write the biochemical basis for the following clinical findings: i. Neurological manifestations ii. Light colored hair and skin iii. Mousy body odor d. Describe the steps for synthesis of any two biological important compounds derived from tyrosine.			
9. Name the sulfur-containing amino acids. Describe in detail the metabolism of essential sulfur-containing amino acid and add a note on the special products synthesized from it. Add a note on inborn errors associated with its pathway.	360	313	D05, D12
10. What is the active form of methionine? How it is formed? What are its function? Enumerate the steps of methionine metabolism. Write the disorders associated with its metabolism.	361	313	J00
Short Essays			
1. What are nitrogen producing substances in the body? Explain how they are excreted from the body.	—	—	D17(RS3)
2. What are transamination reactions? Giving two examples discuss the importance of these reactions.	333	294	J13(RS3), D16(RS3), J06, J11, D15
3. Describe transamination. Mention the clinical significance of serum transaminases.	333	294	J05
4. Name the coenzyme forms of vitamin B_6. Write the mechanism of transamination.	333	339	J01
5. How ammonia is detoxified in the body?	337	295	J06(RS2), J09
6. Urea cycle (urea formation in liver)—steps, regulations, disorders.	338	297	D06(RS2), J07(RS2), D00, D03, D10, D12, D14
7. How is urea synthesized in the body? Give the reactions. What is the significance of urea cycle?	338	297	D13(RS3)
8. Disorders associated with urea cycle.	341	299	D15
9. How is glycine synthesized in the body? Name the products synthesized from glycine (biomedical importance/metabolic role/fate of glycine).	343	307	D06(RS2), D17(RS3), J98, D09, D15

Contd...

BIOCHEMISTRY

Contd...

	STNRN	VSDN	
10. Compounds synthesized from glycine and enumerate the steps of synthesis of creatine.	344	308	J12
11. Pathway for synthesis of creatine, phosphocreatine and creatinine. Clinical significance of creatinine kinase.	345	308	J18(RS3)
12. How creatine phosphate is synthesized? Mention the significance of estimation of urinary creatinine.	345	308	D01
13. How is creatine synthesized? Add a note on creatinine clearance test with respect to it's reference range and significance.	345	308	D11
14. Biochemical importance of phenylalanine.	346	333	J15
15. Is tyrosine an essential amino acid? Justify. Write the reactions of three important biological products formed from tyrosine.	346	333	D12(RS3)
16. List the important products formed from tyrosine and write the metabolic pathways leading to the formation of any two of them.	349	333	D07(RS2)
17. Name and explain the steps of formation of three important compounds formed from tyrosine.	349	333	J14
18. Mention the catecholamines. How are they formed?	349	334	D16(RS3), D03
19. Outline the synthesis of epinephrine and give its functions.	349	334	J15(RS3)
20. What is phenylketonuria (PKU)? What are the alternate metabolic pathways for the accumulated phenylalanine? How is it diagnosed biochemically?	352	336	D09(RS2), D10
21. Discuss phenylketonuria under (i) enzyme defect, (ii) Manifestation, (iii) Diagnostic test.	352	336	D15(RS3)
22. Describe tryptophan metabolism.	355	339	J16(RS3)
23. Serotonin	357	339	J08(RS2), D98, D99
24. Describe the fate and functions of methionine.	361	313	D13(RS3)
25. Explain how S-adenosyl methionine is formed. Give examples of five transmethylation reactions.	361	313	J15

Contd...

Contd...

	STNRN	VSDN	
26. S-adenosyl methionine—formation, functions.	361	313	D00, D09
27. Metabolic functions of methionine.	361	314	D05, D13
28. Transmethylation reactions with examples.	362	314	J09(RS2), J10(RS2), J12(RS3), J12
29. Describe the conversion of methionine to cysteine. Add a note on homocystinuria.	362	313	J15(RS3)
30. Metabolic functions of cysteine.	363	315	J05(RS2)
31. Disorders of sulfur-containing amino acids.	363	317	D08(RS2)
32. Cystinuria and homocystinurias.	363	317	J11
33. Describe one carbon metabolism. What is its significance?	365	301	D15(RS3), D07
34. Maple syrup urine disease.	367	325	J09(RS2)
35. Write about aminoaciduria.	376	345	J07
36. Name the biochemical defect in the following disorders of amino acid metabolism.	377	346	D01
a. Phenylketonuria.			
b. Alkaptonuria.			
c. Maple syrup urine disease.			
d. Albinism.			
e. Homocystinuria.			
37. Name the enzyme defective in:	340	346	D05
a. Alkaptonuria.	341		
b. Niemann-Pick disease.	341		
c. Albinism.	342		
d. Gaucher's disease.	342		
Short Answers			
1. Significance of non-protein nitrogenous substances.	—	433	J07(RS2)
2. Transamination reaction and clinical importance.	333	294	J09(RS2), D13(RS3)
3. Formation of ammonia and its toxicity in brain.	336	294	D09(RS2)
4. Formation of glutamine and its importance.	337	320	D12

Contd...

Contd...

	STNRN	VSDN	
5. Carbomoyl phosphate synthetase deficiency.	342	299	J98
6. What is the normal level of non-protein nitrogen (NPN) substances in the blood?	342	433	J08
7. Specialized/biologically important compounds formed from glycine.	344	308	D18(RS3), D19(RS3), D03, J13, D14
8. How is creatinine synthesized?	345	308	J15, D16
9. Name the amino acid used for the synthesis of creatinine.	345	308	J07
10. Biologically important compounds derived from tyrosine.	349	333	D08(RS2), J11, D11
11. Melanin synthesis.	349	333	D15
12. Phenylketonuria.	352	336	D00
13. Indicate the biochemical defect in phenylketonuria.	352	336	J14
14. Alkaptonuria.	353	337	D14(RS3), J12, D15
15. Albinism.	354	338	J13
16. Derivatives of tryptophan.	355	339	J12(RS3), D05, D16
17. Serotonin—formation, functions of serotonin.	357	339	D12(RS3), J00, D00
18. Melatonin.	359	341	D15(RS3)
19. Hartnup's disease.	360	342	J12(RS3), J17(RS3), D14
20. Name the sulfur-containing amino acids. List two disorders of their metabolism.	360	313	D02
21. S-adenosyl methionine (active methionine)—formation.	361	313	D98, D11
22. Three transmethylation reactions of S-adenosyl methionine.	362	315	J18(RS3)
23. Homocysteine.	363	293	J09
24. Functions of cysteine.	363	315	D15
25. Enumerate the metabolic disorders associated with cysteine metabolism indicating the defect.	363	317	J02
26. Write the composition of: a. 3-phosphoadenosine-5-phosphosulfate (PAPS) b. S-adenosyl methionine (SAM).	a) 363 b) 361	313	D13

Contd...

Contd...

	STNRN	VSDN	
27. What is meant by inborn error of metabolism? What is homocystinuria?	364	318	D11
28. Maple syrup urine disease.	367	325	J00
29. Name the deficient enzyme in: a. Hyperargininemia b. Phenylketonuria.	368 352	346	J13
30. How GABA is formed? What is its function?	371	336	J03
31. Name the amino acids which form succinyl CoA.	375	319	D06
32. Name two metabolic disorders of amino acids metabolism and indicate the enzyme defect.	377	346	D07
33. Mention the enzyme defects in phenylketonuria and homocystinuria.	377	346	J05
34. Name the enzyme defect in: a. Phenylketonuria b. Alkaptonuria.	377	346	D14
35. Name the biochemical defect in: a. Phenylketonuria b. Maple syrup urine disease.	377	346	J03
36. Polyamines and their clinical significance.	378	324	F21(RS4), D15(RS3)
Multiple Choice Questions			
1. The following compounds are biosynthesized by glycine, *except*: a. Creatinine b. Heme c. **Melatonin** d. Purine nucleotide	343	308	J21(RS4)
2. Appearance black color urine is seen in: a. Porphyria b. **Alkaptonuria** c. Jaundice d. Urinary tract infection	353	337	J21(RS4)

CHAPTER 16: INTEGRATION OF METABOLISM

Short Essays			
1. Explain the metabolic adaptations occurring in the liver and adipose tissue in a well-fed state.	384	364	F21(RS4)

Contd...

Contd...

	STNRN	VSDN	
2. Discuss the biochemical/metabolic changes during starvation.	385	365	J14(RS3), J03, J13, D14
Short Answers			
1. Sources and fate of acetyl CoA.	—	—	D01, J12
2. Biochemical changes in starvation.	385	365	J16(RS3)

CHAPTER 17: METABOLISM OF NUCLEOTIDES

Long Essays			
1. What are nucleotides? Explain the catabolism of purine nucleotides. Write briefly on the metabolic disorders associated with purine metabolism.	72, 395	617, 624, 625	J07(RS2)
2. What are sources of C and N atoms of purine? Describe the biosynthesis of purine and add a note on its regulation.	389	620	J13(RS3)
3. Enumerate the reactions of purine degradation and add a note on gout.	395	624, 625	J13
4. How is uric acid formed from purine and add a note on hyperuricemia.	395	624, 625	J18(RS3)
5. Describe the synthesis of pyrimidine and its regulation.	399	627	D12(RS3)
Short Essays			
1. What are nucleotides? What are the sources of C and N atoms of purine nucleotide? Mention the metabolic disorders associated with purine metabolism.	72, 389, 399	617	J14(RS3)
2. Briefly outline the steps of de novo synthesis of purine.	391	620	D11(RS3), J12(RS3)
3. Purine salvage pathways.	393	624	D06(RS2), J15(RS3), D08, J11, D13, D14
4. Salvage pathway.	393, 402	624	J12(RS3), D05(RS2)
5. Catabolism (degradation) of purines, nucleotides and related disorders (causes of hyperuricemia).	395	624	D06(RS2), D09(RS2), D10(RS2), D13(RS3), D19(RS3), D09, J11
6. Explain the disorders associated with purine synthesis and breakdown.	395	625	F21(RS4)

Contd...

Contd...

	STNRN	VSDN	
7. Synthesis of uric acid.	395	624	J98
8. How is uric acid formed in the body? What is gout? What is the treatment? Explain the basis for the treatment.	395	624	D15(RS3)
9. Hyperuricemia—causes, features and drugs to lower plasma uric acid levels	395	625	J04, J10
10. What is gout? Give its biochemical basis, clinical manifestations and line of treatment.	395	625	D12(RS3), D16(RS3), D99, D00, D07, D11
11. Lesch-Nyhan syndrome and orotic aciduria.	399, 402	626, 629	J05(RS2), D08(RS2)
12. A 4-year-old child was brought to the hospital with the following complaints developmental failure, aggressive behavior, joint pain, compulsive urge to bite his lips and fingers. Mother revealed a family history of similar illness among family members. a. Suggest the probable diagnosis. b. Name an appropriate biochemical parameter to diagnose this condition and state its reference range in males and females. c. Name the enzyme deficiency and the reaction catalyzed by the enzyme.	399	626	J21(RS4)
13. Degradation of pyrimidines.	402	630	J08(RS2)
Short Answers			
1. Indicate sources of various (carbon and nitrogen) atoms of purine ring by a diagrammatic representation.	389	620	J21(RS4), D09(RS2), D03, D07
2. Describe two reactions of salvage pathway of purine nucleotide synthesis.	393	624	J05
3. What is the function of thioredoxin?	394	629	D09
4. Hypoxanthine.	395	624	D98
5. Mention any two causes of hyperuricemia.	395	625	J06
6. Gout—causes.	395	625	J05(RS2), D01
7. What is the normal serum uric acid level? Name two pathological conditions associated with hyperuricemia.	395	625	D02
8. Allopurinol.	398	625	J98
9. Lesch-Nyhan syndrome—causes, features.	399	626	J10(RS2), D14(RS3), D03, J08, J15

Contd...

Contd...

	STNRN	VSDN	
10. Mention the sources of carbon and nitrogen atoms of pyrimidine bases.	400	627	F21(RS4), D13
11. Deficiency features of orotic aciduria. Explain the biochemical basis of manifestations (causes).	402	629	J11(RS2), D19(RS3), J07, J10, D16

CHAPTER 18: MINERAL METABOLISM

Long Essays

	STNRN	VSDN	
1. Describe in detail the sources, daily requirement, absorption, distribution, functions, normal level and factors regulating blood calcium level. Discuss about any clinical condition with abnormal blood calcium level (tetany).	406	559	D06(RS2), J09(RS2), D00, D01, J12, D14
2. A 12-year-old girl presented with stiffness and tingling of hands and feet, carpopedal spasm. On examination, Trousseau's sign was positive, Chvostek sign was positive. On laboratory evaluation, serum calcium was significantly reduced. a. Interpret the findings and suggest the probable diagnosis. b. Mention the reference range and dietary sources of the nutrient. c. Explain the role of hormones in regulating the blood levels of this nutrient. d. Mention any six biochemical functions of this nutrient.	411	564	F21(RS4)
3. Explain the metabolism of iron under the following headings. (a) Absorption and transport, (b) Biochemical functions, (c) Hemosiderosis.	416	567	D13

Short Essays

	STNRN	VSDN	
1. List any three trace elements with their biological function.	407	559	J17(RS3)
2. Calcium—sources, daily requirements, factors affecting absorption, biochemical role (functions) and deficiency signs of calcium.	406	559	J12(RS3), J98, D99, D03, J09, D11
3. Intestinal absorption of calcium.	408	560	J15
4. Calcium homeostasis (regulation of blood calcium level)—by vitamin D, PTH and calcitonin.	409	561	D09(RS2), J00, J02, D07, D13

Contd...

Contd...

	STNRN	VSDN	
5. Write briefly about the role of parathyroid hormone in the regulations of serum calcium level.	409	562	J06
6. Renal rickets.	411	—	J98
7. Give an account of phosphorus metabolism.	412	566	J13(RS3)
8. What are the major biochemical functions of sodium and potassium? Mention their normal serum levels.	413, 414	482, 484	D12(RS3), D03
9. What is the normal range of serum potassium and write about hypokalemia.	414	484	D10(RS2)
10. Iron—source, daily requirement, absorption, factors affecting iron absorption, transports, storage and physiological role of iron.	416	567	J07(RS2), D12(RS3), D16(RS3), D98, D99, D02, J04, J07, J10, J13, D15
11. A 13-year-old girl complains of excessive tiredness, poor appetite and tingling sensation in the limbs. On examination she was pale. Laboratory report revealed Hb—7 g/dL, TIBC is increased, serum transfer in saturation is reduced and peripheral smear showed microcytic hypochromic anemia. a. Suggest the probable diagnosis. b. Describe the absorption and transport of this nutrient.	418	572	J21(RS4)
12. What are the causes and consequences of iron toxicity?	419	573	D16
13. What is Wilson's disease? State the cause and treatment policy.	420	575	D17(RS3)
14. Functions of iodine.	420	575	J11(RS2)
15. Functions of selenium.	423	576	J10 (RS2)
Short Answers			
1. List routinely measured serum electrolytes. Mention their reference range.	—	480	F21(RS4)
2. What is renal tubular acidosis? Mention two biochemical findings in this condition.	—	—	J02
3. Trace elements.	405	559	D06(RS2), D08(RS2)
4. Functions of calcium.	406	560	J11, D16

Contd...

Contd...

	STNRN	VSDN	
5. What is the normal serum calcium level? Explain its regulation.	409	561	D05(RS2), J05
6. List the hormones in plasma calcium regulation.	409	561	D06
7. Calcitriol.	409	561	J98
8. Write short note on rickets.	411	—	J13
9. Functions of magnesium.	412	464	J09
10. Hyponatremia (causes).	414	483	J98
11. Write the normal biological reference value for serum potassium. Mention any two causes of hyperkalemia.	414	484	J21(RS4)
12. Describe the functions of potassium.	414	484	J05
13. Iron—absorption, transport and storage. Add a note on hemochromatosis.	417	568	D10(RS2), D19(RS3), D00, D10
14. Ferritin.	418	569	D08
15. What is hemosiderosis? How it is caused?	419	573	
16. Causes of hemochromatosis.	419	573	J01, D04
17. Functions of copper.	419	574	J12(RS3), N20(RS3), D09
18. Copper-containing protein and its clinical significance.	419	574	J98
19. Four enzymes with copper as integral component.	419	574	D12(RS3), J02, D08
20. Menke's disease.	420	574	J12(RS3)
21. Wilson's disease.	420	574	J00
22. Importance of iodine.	420	575	J14(RS3)
23. Iodine metabolism.	421	681	D07(RS2)
24. Biological role of zinc in the body.	421	575	J06(RS2), D98, J99, J08, J10, J12, J14
25. Name a zinc-containing enzyme and its catalytic role.	421	575	D05
26. Fluorosis.	423	576	J08(RS2)
27. Functions of fluoride in dental health.	423	575	J07
28. Metabolic role of selenium.	423	576	J18(RS3), D99, D08, J15
29. Mention the functions of (a) Iodine, (b) Zinc.	420, 421	575	D01

Contd...

Contd...

	STNRN	VSDN	
30. Describe the functions of iodine and fluorine.	420, 423	575	J05
31. Functions (metabolic roles) of zinc and selenium.	421, 423	575, 576	J05(RS2), J01, D04
Multiple Choice Questions			
1. ______________ is the marker of bone formation. a. Telopeptides b. Tartrate resistant acid phosphatase c. **Osteocalcin** d. Pyridinium cross-links derived from collagen	—	565	J21(RS4)

SECTION 4: CLINICAL BIOCHEMISTRY AND NUTRITION

CHAPTER 19: HORMONES

Short Essays			
1. General mechanism of action of steroid hormones.	430	811	J08(RS2)
2. Give a diagrammatic representation of mechanism of steroid hormone action.	432	811	D12(RS3)
3. Significance of aldosterone.	444	815	J99, D04
Short Answers			
1. Thyroid function tests—routine and anti-thyroid peroxidase antibody (TPO).	—	818	D11(RS3)
2. What is second messenger? Give an example.	430	804	D11
3. Mechanism of action of steroid hormones.	430	811	D14(RS3)
4. Give a diagrammatic representation of action of a steroid hormone.	432	811	J05
5. Cyclic AMP—functions.	432	804	D03
6. Reference range of TSH and its significance.	442	819	D11
7. Clinical interpretation of estimation of thyroid stimulating hormone (TSH) in blood.	442	819	D09(RS2)
8. Laboratory diagnosis for hypothyroidism.	443	818	J16(RS3)

Contd...

Contd...

	STNRN	VSDN	

CHAPTER 20: ORGAN FUNCTION TEST

Short Essays

1. Liver function tests—classify, describe tests based on secretary/metabolic and excretory functions.	454	415	D08(RS2), J14(RS3), D19(RS3), J98, J01, D03, J06, J10, D10, J11
2. Vander Bergh's reaction (principle) and its clinical significance.	456	416	D00, J13, J15
3. Serum enzymes estimated to access the liver function.	456	417	D98
4. Hippuric acid test.	460	—	D15
5. Describe renal function tests. Explain the principle and application of creatinine clearance.	460	429	F21(RS4), J02, J05
6. Explain the tests done to assess the renal tubular functions? What is urine osmolality? Write is reference range.	461	439	J21(RS4)
7. Clearance tests.	462	433	J06(RS2), J15
8. Define renal clearance. Name clearance tests used to asses kidney function. Explain any one of the clearance tests and mention its significance.	462	433	D05(RS2)
9. Creatinine clearance test.	462	434	D08
10. Standard urea clearance test.	463	436	J12(RS3)
11. Concentration dilution test.	463	439	D15

Short Answers

1. Test for urobilinogen.	—	417	J99
2. Enumerate three/four functions of the liver and tests with reference ranges to assess them.	455	415	D11(RS3), D07
3. Describe Vander Bergh's reaction. Mention its significance.	456	416	J18(RS3), D18(RS3), J99, J04, D14
4. Write short note on enzyme assays for liver function/Marker enzymes of liver function test.	456	417	D16(RS3), D13
5. Enumerate renal function tests.	460	429	J11(RS2), D03
6. Tests to assess renal tubular function.	461	439	J17(RS3)
7. Tests of renal distal tubular function.	—	439	J16(RS3)

Contd...

Contd...

	STNRN	VSDN	
8. What is meant by renal clearance? How is creatinine clearance calculated?	462	433	D14(RS3)
9. Clearance tests.	462	433	D06(RS2), N20(RS3)
10. Creatinine clearance test.	462	434	J09(RS2), J13(RS3), D14
11. Alkaline tide.	465	432	D98

CHAPTER 21: WATER, ELECTROLYTE AND ACID-BASE BALANCE

Long Essays

1. What is the normal pH of blood? Explain the mechanism of how it is regulated.	475	461	J12(RS3)
2. What is the normal range of blood pH? What is the importance of maintaining acid-base balance in the body? Write in detail how kidney helps in maintaining acid-base balance. Add a note on metabolic acidosis	475, 483	461, 462, 470	D07(RS2), N20(RS3)

Short Essays

1. Discuss the regulation of water by rennin-angiotensin system.	—	463	D17(RS3)
2. Define pH and buffer. Mention the buffer systems present in plasma, erythrocytes and urine.	476	460	J02
3. What are buffers? Name the buffer system of body fluids. Discuss any one/two buffer system of the body.	476	460	D05(RS2), J13(RS3)
4. What are buffers? Explain the plasma buffers in maintaining acid-base balance.	476	460	J16(RS3), D18(RS3)
5. Blood buffers and their role in acid-base balance.	476	460	J06(RS2), D99, J06
6. Extracellular buffers.	476	460	J10(RS2)
7. Bicarbonate buffer system of blood.	476	460	J09(RS2)
8. What is Henderson-Hasselbach equation? Describe the buffer systems in blood and urine.	477	461	J05
9. Write the Henderson-Hasselbach equation and its significance in bicarbonate buffer system.	477	461	J14(RS3)
10. Use of phosphate buffer in maintaining acid-base balance.	477	461	D10

Contd...

BIOCHEMISTRY

Contd...

	STNRN	VSDN	
11. Renal regulation and respiratory regulation of body pH.	477	463	D00, D01, D03
12. Role of lungs in pH maintenance (respiratory regulation of pH).	477	462	D08
13. Erythrocytes in acid-base balance.	478	463	J18(RS3)
14. Chloride shift.	478	—	J08(RS2)
15. Renal regulation of acid-base balance (give the key reactions of renal mechanism in acid-base balance).	478	463	D06(RS2), D09(RS2), D11(RS3), D12(RS3), J15(RS3), J09, J12, J14, D14
16. Name the urinary buffers. Explain their role in excreting excess acid from the body. Mention the other renal mechanisms of pH homeostasis.	478	463	J21(RS4)
17. What is anion gap? Explain normal anion gap acidosis and high anion gap acidosis with examples.	482	468	J05(RS2), D10(RS2), D09
18. Write the formula to calculate anion gap. Mention its reference range. Discuss the clinical use of anion gap in classifying metabolic acidosis with two examples for each type.	482	468	J21(RS4)
19. What is metabolic alkalosis? Mention four causes of metabolic alkalosis. Explain the compensatory mechanism.	483	470	F21(RS4)
20. How does metabolic alkalosis differ from respiratory alkalosis. Explain the cause and compensatory mechanism involved?	483	470, 471	J00
21. Metabolic acidosis—primary defect, causes, biochemical findings.	483	468	J08(RS2), J19(RS3), D19(RS3), J98, J11
22. Explain metabolic and respiratory acidosis.	483	468, 471	J07(RS2)
23. What are the causes of respiratory acidosis? List the primary abnormalities of respiratory acidosis.	483	471	D14(RS3), J01
24. Respiratory alkalosis.	484	471	D15(RS3)
25. Hormonal regulation of fluid and electrolyte.	470, 473	479	D11(RS3), D16
26. What are buffers? Explain the role of the kidneys in homeostasis of pH of blood.	476, 478	460, 463	D11

Contd...

Contd...

	STNRN	VSDN	
Short Answers			
1. Hormones that regulate water balance.	470	479	J15(RS3)
2. Name the serum electrolytes and give their normal values.	472	478	D01
3. Define buffers. Name the blood buffer system.	476	460	J00, J01, D04, J08, D14
4. What are buffers? Write the importance of bicarbonate buffer system?	476	460	D13, J15
5. Name the most effective physiological buffer in the plasma. Explain the role of carbonic anhydrase in acid-base homeostasis.	476	460	F21(RS4)
6. List the major kidney mechanism for regulation of pH of extracellular fluid.	478	463	D09
7. Carbonic anhydrase.	478	463	D99, D15
8. Discuss the role of carbonic anhydrase in the acid-base regulation.	478	463	D17(RS3)
9. Chloride bicarbonate shift.	478	—	D98
10. Reclamation of bicarbonate by kidneys.	479	462	J01, D04
11. Titratable acidity.	479	463	J99, D99
12. Give an account of anion gap.	482	468	J14
13. What is anion gap? Mention two causes for increased anion gap?	482	468	J03
14. Define anion gap. What happens to anion gap in acidosis resulting from renal failure?	482	468	J07
15. Metabolic acidosis—causes and features	483	468	J04
16. Respiratory acidosis—define, causes, compensation.	483	471	J10, D13
17. Alkalosis.	483	470	D16(RS3)
18. Explain why acidosis causes hyperkalemia? How it is corrected?	484	469	J03
CHAPTER 22: TISSUE PROTEINS AND BODY FLUIDS			
Short Answers			
1. Name any four proteins of the extracellular matrix. Write the post-translational modification of collagen and its importance.	487	785	J21(RS4)
2. Explain the structure of collagen.	488	786	F21(RS4)
3. Amino acids in collagen.	488	786	D99
4. Discuss the nutritional role of milk and dairy products.	495	488	D17(RS3)

Contd...

	STNRN	VSDN	
Multiple Choice Questions			
1. Ehlers-Danlos syndrome is due to the defective formation of: a. Type I collagen b. Type II collagen c. **Type III collagen** d. Type IV collagen	489	788	J21(RS4)
CHAPTER 23: NUTRITION			
Short Essays			
1. What is calorific value? Calculate the energy requirement of a 50-year-old moderate worker.	501	583	F21(RS4)
2. Basal metabolic rate (BMR)—definition, determination, normal value, factors affecting.	502	584	J06(RS2), D07(RS2), J09(RS2), D13(RS3), J18(RS3), D18(RS3), J19(RS3), J08, J09, J12
3. What are dietary fibers? List any four and write their functions. What is meant by dietary fiber? What are the sources of dietary fibers? Discuss the importance of it in nutrition. Outline the functions of proteins.	507	586	J21(RS4), D14(RS3), J15(RS3)
4. Nitrogen balance—factors affecting.	509	588	J05(RS2), J11(RS2)
5. Define biological value of protein. What do you mean by complementary proteins? Give examples. What is the requirement of protein in diet?	511	588	J17(RS3), J14
6. What is a balanced diet? Discuss the components of a balanced diet.	513	—	J15(RS3), D13
7. Protein-energy malnutrition.	514	590	J10(RS2), D11(RS3), D08
8. Describe the causes and features of kwashiorkor and marasmus.	515	590	J05
9. Name the protein-energy malnutrition disorders. Write important differences between them.	516	590	D19(RS3)
Short Answers			
1. Calorific value—definition, calorific value of protein and fat.	501	583	D02

Contd...

Contd...

	STNRN	VSDN	
2. Respiratory quotient (RQ)—definition, RQ values of carbohydrate, lipids and proteins, factor affecting, conditions associated with lowering RQ.	501	583	J10(RS2), D01, J04, J05, D05, D10, D14, D15
3. Basal metabolic rate (BMR)—definition, factors affecting, causes of increased BMR.	502	584	J02, J04, D09, J10
4. Specific dynamic action (SDA) and basal metabolic rate (BMR).	502	584	D12(RS3)
5. Specific dynamic action of food stuff.	503	585	J12(RS3), J15(RS3), J16(RS3), D07, D12, J15
6. Calculate energy requirement per day of a student of 20 years.	504	585	J13
7. Dietary fiber—sources, examples, beneficial effects (role in health and disease).	507	586	D07(RS2), D08(RS2), J10(RS2), D10(RS2), D18(RS3), J00, J01, J02, D04, D10, J13
8. Define nitrogen balance. Give one example each for conditions with positive and negative nitrogen balance.	509	588	J21(RS4), D10, D11
9. Positive nitrogen balance.	510	588	D10
10. Biological value of protein.	511	588	J15
11. Limiting amino acid.	512	590	J08(RS2)
12. Mutual supplementation of cereals and pulses is beneficial. Justify.	512	593	F21(RS4)
13. Balanced diet.	513	—	J16(RS3), J98, D99, D13
14. Nutritional deficiency disorders in India.	514	589	D07
15. Protein-energy malnutrition (biochemical changes).	514	590	J07(RS2), D10(RS2), D16(RS3), N20(RS3), J13
16. Kwashiorkor—biochemical findings.	515	590	D02, D15
17. Marasmus.	515	590	D98, J06
18. Nutritional deficiency anemias.	515	597	D05(RS2)
19. List two differences between marasmus and kwashiorkor.	516	591	D01

Contd...

Contd...

	STNRN	VSDN	
SECTION 5: MOLECULAR BIOLOGY AND BIOTECHNOLOGY			
CHAPTER 24: DNA—REPLICATION, RECOMBINATION AND REPAIR			
Long Essays			
1. Discuss the structure and replication of DNA.	76, 524	635, 639	J10(RS2)
2. Describe the synthesis of DNA. Write a note on replication of DNA.	524	639	D15(RS3)
3. Define replication. Describe in detail the process of replication in eukaryotes. Mention its inhibitors.	527	639	D14(RS3), J16(RS3)
4. Write about DNA replication and repair.	524, 535	639, 644	J13
Short Essays			
1. What is meant by exonucleases and endonucleases? Write the importance of each.	—	—	J01
2. What is replication? Describe the steps of replication.	524	639	D00, D02, D07
3. Describe the replication of DNA.	527	639	J05
4. Replication of lagging strand.	528	642	D07(RS2)
5. Mutations.	534	646	J05(RS2), N20(RS3)
6. Point mutation—define and effects.	534	—	D17(RS3)
7. Base excision DNA repair mechanism.	536	646	J10
Short Answers			
1. Name bacterial DNA polymerases. Mention its significance.	—	641	D05(RS2)
2. Replication of DNA—any three salient features.	524	639	J21(RS4), D98, J09
3. What is meant by semiconservative mechanism of replication?	524	639	J10
4. Okazaki fragments.	525	642	J17(RS3), D18(RS3), J15, D16
5. Cell cycle.	530	644	J17(RS3)
6. Telomerase are involved in aging process. Justify and give its clinical significance	532	647	J21(RS4)
7. What is mutation? List two examples.	534	646	J02, D14
8. Mutagens.	534	678	J17(RS3)
9. Point mutation with two examples.	534	—	J15(RS3), D15(RS3), J12

Contd...

Contd...

	STNRN	VSDN	
10. Silent mutation.	534	678	J15
11. Missense mutation—list the effects.	535	678	J10, D15
12. What is nucleotide excision repair?	536	646	J07
13. Causes for xeroderma pigmentosa.	536	646	D12(RS3)
Multiple Choice Questions			
1. Helicase enzyme in DNA replication: a. **Unwinds the DNA** b. Releases the supercoils c. Breaks the strands d. Seals the strands	525	641	J21(RS4)

CHAPTER 25: TRANSCRIPTION AND TRANSLATION

Long Essays			
1. Explain the steps of initiation, elongation and termination of transcription (in prokaryotes). How is it regulated? Name the inhibitors of transcription. Add a note on post-transcriptional modification of RNA.	543, 544, 545	652, 654, 657	F21(RS4), D19(RS3), J14
2. Define translation (protein biosynthesis). Describe the steps of translation. Name four inhibitors and their action.	546, 549, 555	660, 665	J14(RS3), J17(RS3)
3. Write in detail the process of translation- in eukaryotes. Add a note on post translational modifications and its inhibitors.	549, 557	660, 665	D18(RS3), J19(RS3)
4. What is genetic code? Describe the process of eukaryotic translation.	546	659, 660	J11(RS2)
5. What is lac-operon? Explain the steps of activation, initiation, elongation and termination of protein biosynthesis and its regulation.	550, 562	657, 684	J05(RS2), D08(RS2), D10(RS2), D11
Short Essays			
1. Transcription (factors required).	540	652	D06(RS2), D01, J06
2. Post-transcriptional modifications of mRNA.	544	654	D09(RS2), D16(RS3), J10, D12
3. Genetic code—definition (Codon), salient features, initiating and terminating codon.	546	659	D06(RS2), J08(RS2), J17(RS3), D17(RS3), D03, J15

Contd...

Contd...

	STNRN	VSDN	
4. Write part played by ribosomes in proteins biosynthesis.	549	658	J00
5. Post-translational modification.	557	654	D15
Short Answers			
1. RNA polymerase.	543	653	D16(RS3), D15
2. Name the post-transcriptional modifications of m-RNA.	544	654	D06
3. Name two inhibitors of RNA synthesis.	545	657	D05
4. Reverse transcriptase and its significance.	546	657	J01, J03, D04, J06
5. Codon and its characteristics. Name the chain initiating codon and chain terminating codons.	546	659	J99, D99, J05, D07
6. Genetic code—characteristic features.	546	659	F21(RS4), D09(RS2), D10(RS2), D19(RS3)
7. Write short note on codon and 'Wobble hypothesis'.	546, 548	659	D13
8. Degeneracy of codon.	547	659	J01, D04, D09
9. Wobble phenomenon.	548	659	J15
10. Which are inhibitors of protein biosynthesis?	555	657	J07(RS2)
11. Post-translational modifications with examples.	557	654	J13(RS3), D07

CHAPTER 26: REGULATION OF GENE EXPRESSION

Short Essays			
1. Describe with an example regulation of gene expression.	561	683	D13(RS3)
2. Explain Lac operon concept with a diagrammatic representation.	562	684	J21(RS4), D17(RS3), J11
Short Answer			
1. Operon concept.	562	684	D11(RS3)

Contd...

BIOCHEMISTRY

Contd...

	STNRN	VSDN	
CHAPTER 27: RECOMBINANT DNA TECHNOLOGY			
Long Essay			
1. Discuss in detail recombinant DNA technology and its clinical application.	571	690	J08(RS2)
Short Essays			
1. Recombinant DNA technology and its applications.	571	690	D08(RS2), J16(RS3), D16(RS3), J17(RS3), J03, J04, D08, D10, D15
2. What is the difference between endonuclease and restriction endonuclease? Give two examples for endonuclease.	—	691	D15(RS3)
3. What is a restriction endonuclease? Give any two examples with their biomedical importance. Explain their role in recombinant DNA technology.	572	691	J13(RS3), J16(RS3)
4. What is plasmid? What is its application in recombinant DNA technology?	—	691	J07(RS2), J10
5. Explain the principle, requirements, steps of polymerase chain reaction and its application.	579	707	F21(RS4), D14(RS3), D18(RS3), J19(RS3), N20(RS3), J15, D16
Short Answers			
1. What is the difference between endonuclease and restriction endonuclease? Give two examples of restriction endonuclease.	—	691	D08(RS2)
2. What are molecular scissors? Mention its applications.	572	691	F21(RS4)
3. What are restriction enzymes? List three features of restriction enzymes.	—	691	D14(RS3)
4. What is a chimeric (recombinant) DNA molecule? Give the applications of recombinant technology.	572	692	D09(RS2), D11(RS3), D05, D11, D12
5. What are restriction endonucleases? Give two examples.	572	691	D03

Contd...

BIOCHEMISTRY

Contd...

	STNRN	VSDN	
6. What is a vector? What are the commonly used vectors in recombinant DNA technology?	574	691	J18(RS3), J07
7. What is Southern blot technique? Write two applications of this technique.	576	704	J14(RS3)
8. What are DNA probes? Mention the types DNA probes. Write their applications	578	704	J21(RS4), D17(RS3)
9. What is polymerase chain reaction (PCR)? Mention application of PCR.	579	707	J05(RS2), J06(RS2), J09(RS2), J14(RS3), J04
10. What is restriction fragment length polymorphism? Give one clinical application for the same.	583	706	J07
Multiple Choice Questions			
1. Western blot technique is used for the: a. Detection of specific DNA segment b. Detection of specific gene expression c. **Identification of a specific protein** d. Location of a gene on a specific chromosome	577	705	J21(RS4)

SECTION 6: CURRENT TOPICS

CHAPTER 28: HUMAN GENOME PROJECT

None

CHAPTER 29: GENE THERAPY

Short Essay			
1. Gene therapy—its application in medicine.	602	697	D07(RS2), D13(RS3), D09, D12
Short Answer			
1. What is gene therapy? Name vectors used for gene therapy.	602	697	D05(RS2), D18(RS3)
Multiple Choice Questions			
1. Which of the following has not been treated by gene therapy? a. Hemophilia b. Severe combined immunodeficiency c. Cystic fibrosis d. **Glucose-6-phosphatase deficiency**	603	625	J21(RS4)

Contd...

Contd...

	STNRN	VSDN	

CHAPTER 30: BIOINFORMATICS

None

CHAPTER 31: METABOLISM OF XENOBIOTICS (DETOXIFICATION)

Short Essays

1. What are xenobiotics? Give an account of phase two detoxification reactions.	613	505	D18(RS3)
2. What is biotransformation? Discuss the different phases of biotransformation with an example.	613	505	J14(RS3)
3. Detoxification with examples of reactions involved.	613	505	D05(RS2), J05, J13
4. Define detoxification. Give any four reactions of phase II detoxification.	613	505	J17(RS3)
5. What is detoxification? Explain the role of oxidation and conjugation reactions in the liver for detoxification.	613	505	D11
6. Detoxification by oxidation.	614	504	J11(RS2)
7. Detoxification by conjugation with examples.	615	505	D19(RS3), D10

Short Answers

1. How is paracetamol detoxified?	—	—	J08
2. What are xenobiotics? What is the role of Glutathione in detoxification.	613	506	D10(RS2)
3. What is biotransformation? Give two examples.	613	503	D02
4. Detoxification.	613	503	D17(RS3), J11
5. What is detoxification? Give two examples of conjugation phase reactions?	613	503	J21(RS4)
6. Explain any one detoxification mechanism with an example.	614	503	D12
7. Write the process of phase i detoxification with one example.	614	503	F21(RS4), D14(RS3)
8. Give two examples of detoxification by oxidation and reduction.	614	503	D09(RS2)
9. Detoxification of alcohol.	614	504	J09(RS2)
10. Role of cytochrome P450 in detoxification reaction.	615	504	D08(RS2), D14
11. How is aspirin detoxified?	615	505	D07
12. Phase two reactions of detoxification.	615	505	J19(RS3)

Contd...

Contd...

	STNRN	VSDN	
13. Conjugation as detoxification mechanism with two examples.	615	505	J06(RS2), J07(RS2), D98

CHAPTER 32: PROSTAGLANDINS AND RELATED COMPOUNDS

Short Essays

1. What are eicosanoids? Mention their biomedical importance.	618	279	J02
2. Products from arachidonic acid and their function.	618	279	D19(RS3)
3. Prostaglandins—classification and biological action.	620	279	J09(RS2), D98, J07

Short Answers

1. Eicosanoids—names/functions.	618	279	D14(RS3), J08, D16
2. What are prostaglandins? Mention their biological functions.	618	279	D06(RS2), D13(RS3), D01, D10
3. What is arachidonic acid? Mention two uses of arachidonic acid.	619	279	J10

CHAPTER 33: BIOLOGICAL MEMBRANES AND TRANSPORT

Short Essays

1. Cell membrane—fluid mosaic model (with a neat labeled diagram).	623	17	F21(RS4), D09(RS2), D17(RS3), J14
2. Different transport mechanisms across the cell membrane.	624	20	J18(RS3), D09, J11
3. Facilitated diffusion.	625	20	D10
4. Define active transport. Explain the different types of active transport with suitable examples.	626	23	D18(RS3), J15
5. Sodium-potassium pump.	626	23	J10
6. Classify transport mechanisms across cell membranes. Define uniport, symport and antiport. Give an example of each.	627	20	D11(RS3)

Short Answers

1. Cell membrane—functions.	—	17	D07(RS2), J09
2. Describe secondary active transport. Mention one disorder of secondary active transport.	—	23	J05

Contd...

BIOCHEMISTRY

Contd...

	STNRN	VSDN	
3. Write four structural features of cell membrane.	623	17	J13
4. Transport across cell membrane.	624	20	D15(RS3)
5. Define the term active and passive transport.	625	20	J13
6. Active transport across membranes.	626	23	J11(RS2), N20(RS3), D06
7. What is uniport and symport transport system? Give an example.	627	23	D11
8. Endocytosis.	628	25	D08, J11

CHAPTER 34: FREE RADICALS AND ANTIOXIDANTS

Short Essays

1. Classify antioxidants giving two examples for each class.	632	500	J21(RS4), J08(RS2), J99, D04
2. Explain the role of antioxidants in protection against reactive oxygen species (ROS).	632	500	F21(RS4)
3. Antioxidant vitamins.	632	500	D06

Short Answers

1. Free radicals—definition, generation, functions.	629	495	J05(RS2), J12(RS3), D10
2. Reactive oxygen species (ROS)—enumerate, formation, characteristics.	630	495	D08(RS2), D10(RS2)
3. Free radicals and disease.	631	495	J11(RS2)
4. Significance of free radicals and antioxidants.	631	495	N20(RS3)
5. Free radical scavenging systems.	632	497	D18(RS3)
6. Antioxidants with examples.	632	500	D06(RS2), D11(RS3), D12(RS3), J15(RS3), D98, D03
7. What are antioxidants? Name chain breaking and preventive antioxidants.	632	500	J07(RS2)
8. Nonenzymatic antioxidants.	632	500	J16(RS3)
9. Mention the dietary antioxidants.	632	500	J14

Contd...

Contd...

	STNRN	VSDN	

CHAPTER 35: ENVIRONMENTAL BIOCHEMISTRY

Short Answer

	STNRN	VSDN	
1. What are the effects of lead poisoning on heme synthesis?	638	382	J14

CHAPTER 36: INSULIN, GLUCOSEHOMEOSTASIS AND DIABETES MELLITUS

Long Essay

	STNRN	VSDN	
1. What is the normal blood glucose level? Why does it need to be regulated? Describe the regulation of blood glucose. What are the causes of hyperglycemia and hypoglycemia?	646	180	D09(RS2), D14(RS3), D03

Short Essays

	STNRN	VSDN	
1. Regulation of blood sugar.	646	180	D12
2. Mechanisms of action of glucagon.	646	190	D07(RS2)
3. Explain the role of hypoglycemic hormones (insulin) in regulation of blood glucose.	648	186	J05(RS2)
4. Glucose tolerance test (GTT).	652	164	D02, J07, D09
5. Diabetes mellitus (metabolic changes).	654	173	D08(RS2), D12(RS3)

Short Answers

	STNRN	VSDN	
1. Glucose tolerance test (GTT) graph for renal glycosuria.	—	182	D11(RS3)
2. Name two physiological actions of insulin.	643	186	D05
3. Intracellular insulin receptor.	644	168	J06(RS2)
4. What are metabolic effects of glucagon?	645	190	J04
5. How does insulin regulate blood glucose?	648	169	D13
6. Name the insulin antagonists.	648	190	D01
7. Hyperglycemic hormones and their mode of action.	648	190	D19(RS3)
8. Glucose tolerance test.	652	182	J11
9. What are the features of a normal glucose tolerance curve?	652	182	J10
10. Fasting and glucose tolerance test criteria for diagnosis of diabetes of diabetes mellitus.	653	181	J19(RS3)
11. What is glycosuria? Mention the causes of different types of glycosuria.	653	185	J04

Contd...

Contd...

	STNRN	VSDN	
12. Renal threshold for glucose and its significance.	653	184	D10(RS2)
13. Renal glycosuria.	653	184	J10(RS2), J99, J12, J14, J15
14. What is renal glycosuria? How do you differentiate it from diabetic glycosuria?	653	184	J03
15. Explain the rationale behind using glycated hemoglobin (HbA1c) as an indicator of glycemic control in diabetes mellitus. What is the reference range for HbA1c.	655	198	F21(RS4)

CHAPTER 37: CANCER

Short Essays

1. What are oncogenes? Discuss two tumor markers and their clinical application.	659, 662	774	D15(RS3)
2. Proto-oncogenes and oncogenes (mechanisms involved in activation of proto-oncogenes to oncogenes).	660	774	D10(RS2), D16
3. Tumor markers (mention five with their diagnostic importance).	662	779	F21(RS4), J07(RS2)
4. Clinical importance of alpha-fetoprotein (AFP) and prostate-specific antigen (PSA). Give their normal values.	663	779	D12(RS3)
5. Mention any four anticancer drugs and write their mechanism of action.	665	781	J21(RS4)

Short Answers

1. Mechanism of carcinogenesis.	—	—	D09(RS2)
2. Plasmids and oncogenes.	—	774	D13(RS3)
3. Prostate specific antigen (PSA).	—	780	J08(RS2)
4. Carcinogens.	658	771	N20(RS3)
5. Chemical carcinogens.	658	771	D16
6. Oncogenes—definition, examples, role in carcinogenesis.	659	774	J05(RS2), D06(RS2), D11(RS3), D18(RS3), J19(RS3), J04, J06, J09
7. Explain the process of activation of proto-oncogenes to oncogenes.	660	774	F21(RS4)
8. What are oncosupressor genes? Name any two with their mechanism of action.	661	775	J21(RS4)

Contd...

Contd...

	STNRN	VSDN	
9. Growth factors—enumerate, functions, role in carcinogenesis.	661	776	D05(RS2), D07(RS2)
10. Tumor markers—definition, examples, diagnostic significance.	662	779	D08(RS2), D14(RS3), D15(RS3), J18(RS3), D02
11. Anticancer agents.	664	780	D13(RS3)

Multiple Choice Questions

1. Serum alpha fetoprotein level is increased in: a. Multiple myeloma b. Choriocarcinoma c. **Hepatoma** d. Lung cancer	663	779	J21(RS4)

CHAPTER 38: ACQUIRED IMMUNODEFICIENCY SYNDROME

None

SECTION 7: BASICS TO LEARN BIOCHEMISTRY

CHAPTER 39: INTRODUCTION TO BIO-ORGANIC CHEMISTRY

None

CHAPTER 40: OVERVIEW OF BIOPHYSICAL CHEMISTRY

Short Essay

1. Radioactive isotopes of iodine and their clinical application.	685	829	D10(RS2)

Short Answers

1. How does a buffer maintain the pH? Give an example of blood buffer.	679	477	D06
2. Define radioactivity. Name the uses of: a. ^{181}I. b. Co-60.	685	829	D01
3. Radioisotopes and application in medicine.	685	829	D13(RS3), N20(RS3)
4. Mention two isotopes and mention their application in medicine.	685	830	D08(RS2), D03, J07

CHAPTER 41: TOOLS OF BIOCHEMISTRY

Short Essays

1. Chromatography.	687	722	J00
2. Electrophoresis.	690	719	D00

Contd...

Contd...

	STNRN	VSDN	
Short Answers			
1. Principle of chromatography.	688	722	J15
2. Electrophoresis—principle, normal pattern of serum proteins, diagnosis importance.	690	719	D15(RS3), D16(RS3), D03, J10, J12
3. Immunoelectrophoresis.	691	721	J08(RS2)
4. Enzyme-linked immunosorbent assay (ELISA).	695	726	N20(RS3)
5. Monoclonal antibodies.	696	753	J14(RS3)
CHAPTER 42: IMMUNOLOGY			
Long Essay			
1. Explain the immunological basis of vaccine development.	—	755	F21(RS4)
CHAPTER 43: MISCELLANEOUS			
Long Essay			
1. Discuss the significance of multienzyme complexes with respect to carbohydrate and lipid metabolism.	—	—	J06(RS2)
Short Essays			
1. Multienzyme complexes.	—	—	D07
2. How would you explain osteoporosis in following conditions? a. Prolonged use of phenobarbitone. b. Chronic liver or renal disease c. Vitamin D resistant rickets d. Fanconi's syndrome e. Vitamin D dependent rickets type II.	—	—	J01
Short Answers			
1. Give reasons for the following:			F21(RS4)
a. Requirement of thiamine is increased in alcoholics.	a. 140	a. 549	
b. Prescription of folic acid during early pregnancy.	b. 155	b. 541	
2. Give reasons for the following			J21(RS4)
a. Muscle glycogen does not contribute to blood glucose.	a. 263	a. 165	
b. Intake of antimalarial drugs like primaquin in some people causes hemolytic anemia.	b. —	b. 78	
c. Humans cannot synthesize vitamin C.	c. 136	c. 548	

Contd...

Contd...

	STNRN	VSDN	
3. Give reason for the following:			J21(RS4)
a. Restriction enzymes are termed as molecular scissors.	a. 572	a. 691	
b. Changing color of the bruise.	b. —	b. —	
c. Hemolytic jaundice is also called acholuric jaundice.	c. 215	c. —	
4. Give reason for the following:			J21(RS4)
a. Pellagra-like symptoms are seen in Hartnup's disease.	a. 360	a. 341	
b. Glycine does not exhibit optical activity.	b. —	b. —	
c. Proline is an α-helix breaker.	c. 59	c. 39	
5. Barbiturates should be given with caution in chronic alcoholics. Justify.	—	—	F21(RS4)
6. State the advantages of automation in clinical biochemistry laboratory.	—	—	F21(RS4)
7. Indicate the biochemical defect in lactose intolerance and Gilbert's disease.	171, 216	147, 386	D13
8. Name the enzyme defects in the following cases: (1) Refsum's disease, (2) Alkaptonuria.	294, 353	228, 338	D13
9. GABA, PUFA and SAM and their importance.	371, 30, 361	36, 106, 507	J14(RS3)
10. Name two inborn errors of metabolism and the associated enzyme.	377	—	J09
11. Abnormal components of urine.	729	431	D13(RS3)
12. Define proteinuria. Mention a biochemical test to detect proteinuria.	—	432	J14
13. What are G-proteins?	—	803	J14
14. Multienzyme complex.	—	—	D17(RS3)
15. What are cold agglutinins?	—	—	D05
16. What is reference range/values? How is it calculated?	—	—	D07(RS2), J16(RS3), J19(RS3)
17. Achylia gastrica.	—	—	J98
18. Reference range of potassium and albumin in the serum.	—	—	D09

Contd...

Contd...

	STNRN	VSDN	
19. Normal values of: a. Serum creatinine (0.5–1.5 mg/dL). b. Serum amylase (80–180 Somogyi units/dL).	—	—	D99
20. Mention the normal serum values for: a. AST (4–45 IU/L). b. ALT (3–40 IU/L). c. Urea (15–40 mg/dL). d. Creatinine (0.5–1.5 mg/dL).	—	—	J02
21. Normal serum levels of: a. Serum calcium (9-11 mg/dL). b. Serum phosphorus (3-4.5 mg/dL).	—	—	J06, D08
22. Mention the normal levels of: a. Serum protein (6–8g/dL). b. Urea (15–40 mg/dL). c. Creatinine (0.5–1.5mg/dL).	—	—	D06(RS2)
23. Give the normal blood level of the following: a. Fasting blood glucose (70–100 mg/dL). b. Total protein (6–8g/dL). c. Urea (15–40 mg/dL). d. Bicarbonate (24–30 mEq/L). e. Sodium (135–145 mEq/L). f. Potassium (3.5–5 mEq/L).	—	—	J09(RS2)
24. Give the normal values of: a. Fasting blood glucose (70–100 mg/dL). b. Cholesterol (150–200 mg/dL).	—	—	D13
25. Name the normal serum levels of: a. Sodium (135–145 mEq/L). b. Potassium (3.5–5 mEq/L).	—	—	J14
26. Give the normal values of: a. Fasting blood glucose (70–100 mg/dL). b. Blood urea (15–40 mg/dL).	—	—	D14
Multiple Choice Questions			
1. Urine preservatives are used for all the following purposes, *except:* a. Reduce bacterial action b. Minimize chemical decomposition c. **Increase pH** d. Decrease atmospheric oxidation of unstable compounds	—	736	J21(RS4)